QUIT SM(

Guided Sleep Meditation to Overcome Nicotine Addiction, Reduce Stress and Get Smoke-Free in 30 Days with Hypnosis and Positive Affirmations + Stop Smoking Challenge!

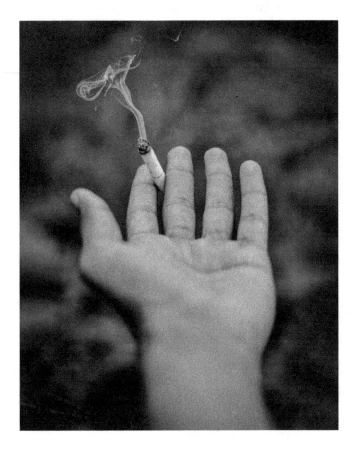

By Elliott J. Power

TABLE OF CONTENTS

Introduction 1

Chapter 1: Trying To Quit Smoking? Here's How Self-Hypnosis Could Help 15

Chapter 2: Hypnosis To Quit Smoking: Does It Work? 25

Chapter 3: Improve Your State Of Mind And Form A Healthy Mindset 34

Chapter 4: Reduce Addiction-Caused Anxiety And Stress 41

How Depression, Anxiety And Addiction Go Together And Why It Matters 51

Chapter 5: Anxiety Disorders And Drug Addiction 58

Anxiety After Drug Use 63

Chapter 6: Ways To Relieve Insomnia When You Quit Smoking 72

Chapter 7: Positive Affirmations To Quit Smoking 78

Chapter 8: Relax And Fall Asleep Easily Every Night 86

Chapter 9: Deep Sleep All Night Long 94

Deep Sleep Requirements 97

Deep Sleep: How To Get More Of It 104

Chapter 10: Calm Your Mind 112

Chapter 11: How Quitting Smoking Has Changed My Life 121

Conclusion 128

Thanks again for choosing this book, make sure to leave a short review on Audible if you enjoy it. I'd really love to hear your thoughts.

INTRODUCTION

Quitting smoking can be very challenging. However, it is one of the best things you can do. Smoking is a dangerous and deadly habit. It's the number one cause of cancer. It also raises the risk of heart attacks, lung disease, strokes and other health problems including cataracts and bone fractures.

If patches, gum chewing, nicotine lozenges, counselling and other forms of smoking cessation have not helped you quit the habit, don't give up. Ask the doctor if hypnosis is an alternative. Some studies have shown that hypnosis can help some people stop smoking.

What is Hypnosis?

Hypnosis is described as an altered state of consciousness where you seem to be asleep or in a trance. Clinical hypnosis can be used to treat some psychological or physical conditions. It's also used to help patients control pain. It's used in a wide variety of other conditions such as weight problems, speech disorders and problems with addictions.

There is a debate on how the hypnosis works. Many people believe you relax and focus more while you're hypnotized, so they're more likely to listen to suggestions — like giving up smoking, for example.

While, during hypnosis, you do appear to be in a trance, you are not unconscious. You're still conscious of your surroundings, and despite what many stage performers may say during an entertainment show — you cannot be forced to do anything against your will.

However, brain tests performed on patients during hypnotism sessions revealed a high degree of neurological activity.

Hypnosis for Smokers

During smoking cessation hypnosis, a patient is often asked to imagine negative smoking outcomes. The hypnotherapist may say, for example, that cigarette smoke smells like truck exhaust, or that smoking may leave the patient's mouth feeling extremely parched.

Spiegel's method is a common technique of hypnosis of smoking cessation, which focuses on three main ideas:

- You need your body to live
- Smoking poisons the body
- You should respect and protect your body (to the extent you'd like to live)

The hypnotherapist advises the smoker to use self-hypnosis, and then tells him or her to reiterate these affirmations if there is a need to smoke.

Does Hypnosis Work?

Hypnosis, in general, doesn't work for everyone. About one in every four people cannot be hypnotized. When successful, the depth of the hypnosis can differ from person to person.

How well the hypnosis works to help people stop smoking depends on who you ask. Results for the study have been mixed. A systematic analysis of scientific research in 2010 revealed that there wasn't adequate evidence to justify the use of hypnosis. Another study released in 2012 said the use of hypnosis offers a potential benefit. The American Cancer Society states in exploring alternative strategies for stopping smoking on its website that while controlled studies have not proven the efficacy of hypnosis, there is anecdotal evidence that certain people have been helped.

Hypnosis is not an approved treatment by the American Medical Association (AMA), despite some websites and promotional materials that suggest otherwise. The organization 's position on using hypnosis is not official. In 1987 the AMA rescinded a consensus statement related to the use of the technique for medical and psychological purposes.

Experts who have researched hypnosis say further, well-conducted research is required to establish if hypnosis helps smokers quit the habit for good, however, adds that hypnosis remains a promising solution and has several other benefits. The best way to quit, however, may be to combine multiple strategies.

How to Find a Hypnotherapist

Ask your healthcare professional to recommend a successful hypnotherapist if you want to try hypnosis to help you stop smoking.

Below are some tips to find a professional hypnotherapist:

- Ensure they are licensed, qualified and certified. Hypnosis for smoking cessation and other medical reasons should only be done by someone with a current license in a field of health care, such as psychiatry, medicine, psychology, or nursing.

- Ask any difficult questions. Ask about the professional training. Also, the American Society for Clinical Hypnosis suggests asking: "Can this practitioner help me without hypnosis? "If the answer is no, look elsewhere then.

- Beware of the claims or promises that are too good to be true. Hypnosis doesn't work for everyone.

It's never too late to stop smoking. Doing so has immediate benefits for health. If you stop smoking before you turn 50, you will cut the risk of dying in the next fifteen years compared to those who keep lighting up.

We have all heard about hypnosis. We've seen the magical practitioners on the adverts promising to liberate us forever from addiction. We've successfully seen Chandler Bing quit smoking just by falling asleep on some tapes calling him strong and confident.

But most of us aren't quite sure what hypnosis is. Where the idea originated from? Is it anything to do with snake-charming? Most importantly: Can it help break a habit of smoking?

I looked into the subject of hypnosis a little deeper, so I can help my readers to distinguish reality from fiction.

The Origins of Hypnosis

In the early 20th century, Sigmund Freud, the founding father of psychoanalysis, brought hypnosis back into the limelight. He wasn't the first to bring up the idea. He was a figurehead also for the role played by hypnosis in modern psychology and medicine.

Freud used hypnosis to help his patients access their unconscious mind to desires and fears. In conversation with the psychoanalyst, patients will enter a trance-like state and allow their deepest feelings to surface. Freud theorized that this would allow them to free up crippling emotions and recover from their anxiety, or hysteria.

Freud was a very bad hypnotist (and smoked like a chimney). Nevertheless, modern health care practitioners have considered Freud 's theories on hypnosis useful. This is because the hypnosis provides a changed state of consciousness. This will allow the subconscious mind to be accessed. The individual will then be able to channel and resolve underlying desires and fears to help them work towards their objectives.

How Hypnosis Works

Experts on hypnosis also provide people with goals to boost their health. Quitting smoking is a common health goal. We all know the advantages of being a non-smoker: healthy skin, higher life expectancy and a greatly reduced risk of lung cancer or heart attack.

You're likely to have some misgivings about the idea of hypnosis and how it works to quit smoking. The thought of getting a stranger induced into a trance is very compelling. You think of this as something entertainers like David Blaine might do to embarrass members of the audience at magic shows.

If you're considering hypnotherapy, I'm here to tell you that Derren Brown won't rock up and trick you into drinking a bottle of vinegar. The goal of professional hypnotherapists is not to make you do things that you don't want. Nevertheless, research shows that hypnosis does not work unless there are existing intentions for the subject to achieve something.

Hypnosis also involves amplifying current wishes-including the need to stop smoking!

So, what would happen during a session of hypnotherapy?

There are many ways to induce hypnosis, none of which includes swinging a watch in front of your eyes (this is a Hollywood myth). The quick movement would be distracting. Hypnosis revolves around concentration.

Hypnotic induction techniques are meant to relax the conscious mind and achieve a trance-like state. The therapists use suggestion and word combinations to have this effect on clients. Hypnotic induction may take place within guided sessions or by using pre-recorded tapes (self-hypnosis).

Entering into a hypnotic trance is not the same as sleeping. It's a very deep state of altered consciousness. Scans have shown that during hypnosis, people generally experience greater brain activity. This increased brain activity is intended to allow an individual to concentrate on their specific goal.

Studies have proposed that some people frequently enter trance-like states. Have you ever been concentrating on a project that you have forgotten lunch? This intense concentration is known as a spontaneous trance, whereas the induction of a hypnotic trance is deeper.

The therapists introduce clients to 'hypnotic suggestions' until they enter a trance. These are statements which promote goals of control, confidence and a smoking-free life.

Often, the client is asked to visualize some things. As a non-smoker, those might be optimistic aspects of a future. They may also be uncomfortable sensations related to current smoking habits.

For these activities, therapists should follow standardized scripts. But sessions on hypnosis can differ a great deal. Hypnosis does not share the same base of evidence as other smoking addictions treatments. This means that approaches like cognitive-behavioral therapy do not have the same proven guidelines.

HYPNOSIS TO QUIT SMOKING – HOW EFFECTIVE IS IT?

Using hypnosis to stop smoking might sound like wishful thinking. However, can you stop smoking for good with the aid of hypnotherapy? In this part of the book, we will discuss the effects on smoking using hypnotherapy, to see whether it brings anything new to the table or not.

The Dangers of Smoking

Smoking causes up to seven million deaths a year, so quitting should be your main priority.

Ditching smoking can be a real challenge. Smoking is a toxic habit that can lead to cancer and death. Although 1.1 billion people around the world are smokers, according to the World Health Organization (WHO). Sadly, many of these smokers come from low- or middle-income countries, and they are suffering from diseases related to tobacco.

The WHO finds the tobacco crisis one of the world's most important challenges to public health. Tobacco consumption is responsible for up to seven million deaths per year. Unfortunately, as many as half of the people who use tobacco die from it.

While most people find it difficult to stop smoking, there are some factors that can help. Lozenges, nicotine patches, and chewing gum will help you conquer your addiction.

However, if you've tried any of these approaches without any success, you don't have to worry. There is still something you can try.

Hypnosis for Smoking

Hypnotherapy is great for helping you break bad habits and deal with stress. Although hypnotherapy is used in a number of ways, it is especially good to relax the mind and help you overcome the risk of relapse.

The History of Hypnosis as a Treatment for Smoking

In the 1950s psychologists started using hypnotherapy as an aid to traditional therapy for psychological care. Back in 1958, hypnotherapy was accepted as a therapeutic treatment by the American Psychological Association (APA) and the American Medical Association (AMA).

Hypnotherapy was first used by Dr Herbert Spiegel to help people stop smoking and was first published in 1970. His treatment technique is well recognized and is still used to this day as the "Spiegel Method."

Modern hypnotherapists use suggestions to encourage smokers to replace tobacco and cigarette smoke with unpleasant feelings that help smokers quit. The hypnotherapists can also improve the ability of smokers to cope with their symptoms of nicotine withdrawal and reduce their urge to smoke.

Hypnosis to Quit Smoking – What Does Science Say?

Hypnosis has always been a controversial topic. People are sceptical about the advantages of hypnotherapy because this alternative medicine branch has been misrepresented for decades in movies and other forms of media. Some people believe that hypnotherapy is nothing but stage magic, while others believe that under the influence of hypnosis, they become more susceptible to suggestion.

However, there are many studies based on the efficacy of the smoking hypnosis. Here are their findings:

1993 Study

A 1993 study looked at the effectiveness of hypnotherapy for smoking cessation. The interesting thing about this study, after a single hypnosis session, is that it studied the effects of hypnotherapy for smokers.

226 Smokers received a single session of hypnosis involving self-hypnosis. Two years after the report, the researchers contacted the smokers to follow up on their findings. This research estimated as a positive outcome only the complete abstinence from smoking.

A week after the hypnosis session, 52 percent of the people who participated in this study abstained from smoking. Over two years, 23 percent of participants maintained their abstinence. Curiously, the study showed that those who lived with a partner were more likely to abstain from smoking than those who did not.

The study found that hypnotherapy was mildly successful in helping people to stop smoking. The researchers discovered that hypnosis is preferable to voluntary efforts to give up smoking.

2008 Study

Research published in May 2008 aimed to determine whether hypnosis would be more effective in helping smokers quit than regular therapy. The randomized research recruited 286 smokers living in San Francisco. The smokers took part in two 60-minute counselling or hypnotherapy sessions, and after the study, they received three follow-up calls.

29 percent of those in the hypnotherapy group indicated abstaining from smoking after seven days into the study, compared to 23 percent in the counseling group.

Six months later, compared to 18 percent of the behavioral treatment group, 26 percent of people who were part of the hypnotherapy group indicated that they did not pick up the habit again.

One year after the study, 20 percent of the hypnotherapy group reported not smoking, compared to just 14 percent of the counselling group.

This research found hypnosis is more effective for long-term quit rates than traditional behavioral therapy.

2014 Study

Research published in 2017 looked at the effectiveness of smoking cessation hypnotherapy among students.

59 Students were randomly chosen to participate in the study. The researchers instructed the students in self-hypnosis techniques, and they asked the students to try it at home and keep a diary of how much they smoked for nine weeks.

The study found that after nine weeks of practicing hypnosis, 65.4 percent of students quit smoking. The study stated that the students smoked less after the program was introduced, and it suggests that hypnotherapy has therapeutic effectiveness in achieving a cessation of smoking among students.

What Makes Hypnosis Effective for Smokers?

So far, we have seen that part of the scientific community supports the use of hypnosis as an aid for those who want to give up smoking. But, why do smokers find hypnosis so effective?

A Different Mindset

Smokers will build a new attitude about cigarettes with the aid of hypnotherapy. The advice from hypnotherapists will make you see cigarettes for what they are.

One of the most common phrases you'll hear when someone tries to quit smoking is that they like to smoke. Well, to give in to your cravings is one thing, and it is another to say that you really like it.

With the aid of suggestions from the hypnotist, the mentality changes. Smoking can no longer be seen as something you want after the therapeutic intervention. You are going to see it as the threat it is. While some of the suggestions may make you nervous at first, they will not only help you stop smoking, but will also help you to conquer your cravings and possible relapses.

Helps You Help Yourself

Most people wrongly think only hypnotherapists can induce hypnosis. This is not true. You can learn to practice self-hypnosis with the aid of a guided therapy session, and help yourself overcome your addiction.

Some words and phrases might help your subconscious view cigarettes differently. Repeating these terms or phrases can help you fight the desire to light a cigarette, and can help you abstain from smoking in the future.

Complementary Method

One of the positive things about hypnotherapy is that to improve the chances of stopping smoking, you can combine it with other approaches. Not only this, hypnotherapy can also improve the effects of certain forms of smoking cessation, such as nicotine patches or chewing gum.

Hypnosis can allow the mind to conquer the addiction while the nicotine gum or patches can allow the body deal with the effects of nicotine withdrawal.

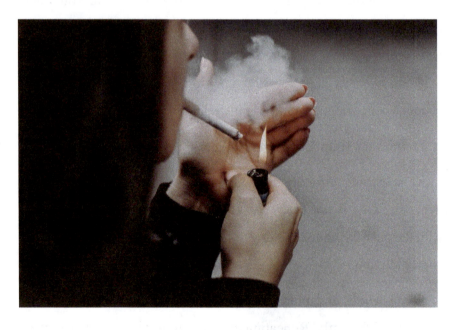

CHAPTER 1
TRYING TO QUIT SMOKING? HERE'S HOW SELF-HYPNOSIS COULD HELP

Want 2020 to be the year you quit smoking for good? According to research from the Change Incorporated Quit Cigarettes mission, more than half (56%) of smokers have tried to quit this month – and more than half (53%) admit they're feeling anxious or nervous about it.

It's not easy to stop smoking. It can be very difficult indeed – but it is possible with the right approach and support. So, if you're still struggling, or have failed previous attempts to quit, maybe it's time to try a new approach?

Smokers are up to four times more likely to quit for good if they use a combination of a medical professional's smoking cessation treatments and support instead of trying to go 'cold turkey.'

Doctor-turned-TV hypnotherapist Aaron Calvert has partnered up with Change Incorporated to help smokers get to the right mindset to quit through self-hypnosis, guided breathing exercises, and mindfulness. Studies show, he points out that you are much more likely to be able to quit for good if you can stay smoke-free for 7 days.

"People who decided to quit smoking cigarettes should feel extremely proud of themselves, because the first thing they should know is that they're not alone," Calvert says. "There are loads of people around the globe planning to quit right now, and I hope the tips and tricks I share make it as easy as possible for people to get through those first 7 days."

Calvert here discusses how to use self-hypnosis to quit smoking, along with several other suggestions to help you keep track of it.

Quitting Through Self-hypnosis,

Self-hypnosis can be used to help you achieve significant changes in your life, such as stopping smoking. Choose your session time and place – make sure it's quiet enough so you won't be interrupted.

Lie down or sit down, and close your eyes. Take three deep, slow breaths and hold the third breath in for three seconds. Relax and sink back into the seat while you breathe out. Concentrate on your breathing, and let your thoughts float in and out as if connected to your breathing until your mind is clear.

Now count backwards from 10 to zero, counting each number as you breathe out and concentrating on a different part of your body, helping it to relax. I begin with my toes and work up to my head, however, you may find that you prefer to do it from your head down to your toes.

You'll be relaxed at this point, but just imagine yourself in a quiet place to help deepen that relaxation. I like using a beach; imagine the beach in as much detail as possible. Try to imagine a meadow or a garden anywhere you feel most comfortable with if you dislike beaches.

Now you're in that state of relaxation and concentration, you can give yourself a suggestion, feel more comfortable about quitting smoking, or imagine your justification for quitting vividly so that you feel more inspired to achieve your goal.

When it's time to wake up, just count yourself all the way back from zero to 10 and you'll find yourself wide awake, feeling refreshed and re-energized. When you need to be immediately awake and alert during your session for some reason, you should be able to wake up, and of course, be yourself. This is it! It's so easy to really start making positive changes in your life.

1. **Text three friends**

If you're tempted to smoke, try texting three friends and wait for their responses before you give in. The urge would have passed by the time they've all replied.

2. **Choose your support network wisely**

Tell your loved ones you are quitting, because they're not only going to support you, they're going to motivate you and provide advice to help you. Also, telling people forces you to be truthful, particularly early on in your journey, as you have someone else to respond to.

3. **Have a plan of action**

Having a plan right from the start means you are more likely to succeed.

4. **Know your reason for quitting**

It's vital, to be honest with yourself – why are you quitting? Is it to save money, enhance your health or the health of those around you, or is it simply to help you look younger or smell better? Whatever the reason, find it, write it down – and put it anywhere you would usually smoke, helping you remember why you're making this positive change.

5. **Reward yourself**

When you fall back into old habits, it's easy to be over-critical of yourself. Slipping up is normal — learn to accept it, and keep on trying to quit. It's equally important to pat yourself on the back when you succeed. Plan to reward yourself when you reach a milestone period of time without smoking — after the vital first seven days, for example, which is worth celebrating.

6. **Stay away from triggers**.

There will be some things in your daily routine that you connect with smoking. It may be a morning coffee, meeting with some friends or during your work break. Avoid your triggers or change your routine for the first few days.

7. **Try straw therapy**

If you are tempted to smoke, you can replace a cigarette with a straw. Cut down a household straw and use it as you would a cigarette. So much smoking is anchored to the hand-to-mouth action, feeling something in your hands and taking a deep breath. This 'straw therapy' can help your body psychologically to stop that craving feeling.

8. **Relax**

Stopping smoking can make you feel more depressed than usual, so make sure you take some extra time out to relax. If you're running, doing some yoga, or using self-hypnosis and relaxation exercises, it's crucial to make sure you stay on top of your game and stay motivated while you quit.

Can You Quit Smoking Through Hypnosis?

"It is all about choice," the man said, with the soothing voice. "If you are here for someone else's pleasure, you can hang around and have some fun, but more than likely you'll go out and smoke after."

I was sitting in the basement of the public library in Arlington, Massachusetts, with a motley group of about 20, we were all skeptical and desperate, with one major thing in common: We smelled like an ashtray.

Theoretically, we should have come together because we no longer wanted to smoke cigarettes. "I am here for health reasons," said one lady. "Cigarettes are too expensive," said an elderly man.

"I am at dental hygiene school," another attendee added. "We should be promoting health, but how can I advise anyone else to quit smoking if I am myself?"

These are positive reasons people would want to stop smoking. It is the same for me, plus vanity, and, the grim specter of an earlier grave. (When you're gone, you can't look good.) So, if I really wanted to stop, why was the only thing I could think of was how much I wanted to go out and smoke a cigarette?

Mark Hall, a qualified hypnotherapist and licensed social worker, knows only too well. He stopped smoking himself several years ago — he says he still recalls reaching for a phantom lighter that wasn't in his pocket — and he's been having these sessions for over twenty years, with the intention of inspiring others that they can do it themselves.

His hypnotherapy sessions usually cost around $150, or $95 with insurance coverage, but this event, funded by the Sanborn Foundation for the Treatment of Cancer, was close to my house and open to the public. In other words, there was no excuse not to go, except maybe a question that had terrified me as the meeting challenged me all week: What if it didn't work? Or, maybe even worse: What if it does? Then what the hell do I do? Smoking is such a big part of my daily life, ridiculous as it sounds, the thought of losing it is disturbing.

Hall asked, "Does anyone here feel like cigarettes are their best friend?" Telling us to clap our hands, then clap them again, leading this time with the opposite hand to one we'd been used to. Everything felt different. Throughout the room, the tone also changed noticeably. "The point," Hall said, "was that, by muscle memory, smoking is a habit that we all do as involuntarily as the way we choose to clap our hands."

People can undergo hypnosis to tackle all kinds of issues — from addictions like mine to emotional trauma. There's some evidence that it may be an effective tool in treating eating disorders, dentistry, and post-traumatic stress disorder, and dealing with birth pain. But there is still enough uncertainty about what it really is given its prevalence, often even among those who have already committed to it. I definitely had no idea what I was in for because I was sitting in my superlatively uncomfortable chair, ready for something, okay. Or maybe nothing.

Hypnotism is such an amorphous concept that when I asked a couple of practitioners what it is, they spend a great portion of the discussion telling me what it is not. Most of us are familiar with the hypnosis process from the well-known stage hypnotist, where guests are picked up from the audience of the nightclub to go through humiliation on stage. Or, if not, then smugly tossing a stopwatch in front of a patient's face from fictional depictions of a Freudian type. These are both major misconceptions; Hall explained as he preps his crowd for the descent into a state of enhanced relaxation.

"My hypnosis is a therapeutic tool and not entertainment," he said, starting to make us feel at ease. But, he joked, "If you told someone you're going to be here tonight, I'll advise you to go home and start clucking like a chicken."

The practice today typically traces its origins back to the 1840s, when Scottish surgeon James Braid built on the notion of what he called "nervous sleep" or, more precisely, "the induction of a state of abstraction or mental concentration in which, as in reverie or unconscious abstraction, the forces of the mind are so profoundly engrossed with a single concept or stream of thought to render the individual unconscious of, or indifferently conscious to, all other ideas, or trains of thought, or impressions."

But, according to the hypnotist and author Charles Tebbutts, confusing hypnosis with sleep (the term is derived from the Greek for sleep), is incorrect as expressed by his student C. Roy Hunter: Mastering Basic Techniques in his book The Art of Hypnosis. Hypnotism, "is in reality a natural state of mind, and is usually induced much more often in daily life than is artificially induced. We are in a natural hypnotic trance every time we get immersed in a novel or a motion picture," Tebetts wrote. Hunter argues that claiming that hypnosis is simply self-hypnosis is more accurate. The hypnotherapist, much like a physical trainer, merely helps the subject persuade themselves to do something they were already able to do, nudging them in the right direction.

Although there is a broad range of methods and types of hypnotism practiced today — something that further confuses our ability to understand it critically or to research it scientifically —

one thing they seem to have in common is an emphasis on relaxation, concentration, harnessing a desire to improve within the person, and creating verbal and visual connections between emotions.

As explained by the American Association of Professional Hypnotherapists: "Hypnosis is just a condition of relaxed concentration. It's a natural state. -- each of us usually enters such a state — sometimes called a trance state — at least twice a day: once when we fall asleep, and once when we wake up."

Hypnotherapists claim they make this cycle simpler, but without the sleeping part. Joseph P. Green and Steven Jay Lynn reviewed 56 studies on the outcomes of smoking cessation hypnosis in a 2000 study for the International Journal of Clinical and Experimental Hypnosis. Although it has usually been shown to be a better choice than no therapy at all, several studies combine hypnosis with other therapeutic approaches, making it difficult to isolate its effects.

It is rare that people try to stop smoking by hypnosis alone, so no two practices are the same, which explains why it is difficult to know if it works.

Moshe Torem, a psychology professor at Northeast Ohio Medical University and the president of the American Society of Clinical Hypnosis, one of many such professional organizations around the country, explained to me the components of the typical hypnotherapist process.

"Hypnosis is a different state of mind coupled with four main characteristics," he said. First is a "highly focused attention on something." It could be a problem that you have, or a problem that you want to address. Second, the subject disassociates themselves from the immediate physical environment. "In the middle of a Boston winter, you focus on the beach in Florida," he said, completely predicting my particular winter-addled frame of mind. "You're going there with your head, instead of driving, and you're completely focused on the beach."

Maybe a nice place to smoke a cigarette.

The third element is that of suggestibility. The person is more receptive to suggestions that he or she has provided. Fourth is what he terms "involuntariness," which means that when you come out of hypnosis, you believe subjectively you have done nothing but that you have achieved everything. For example, you may know that you are being asked to raise your arm, but you feel as though it is being raised by some outside force. Which makes sense, because I am driven by similar subconscious impulses when I reach for a cigarette, particularly when I know I do not need it.

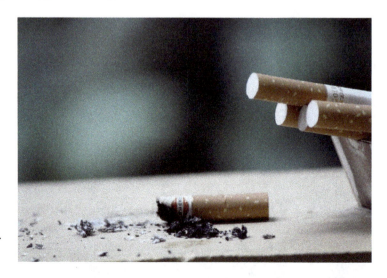

CHAPTER 2
HYPNOSIS TO QUIT SMOKING: DOES IT WORK?

Most smokers get hooked on a habit they hate. This is true. The majority of smokers- an estimated 80%, will be happy to never smoke another cigarette again.

It makes sense too.

We all know smoking is detrimental to your health, moderate smokers felt a sore throat or breathing difficulty as they climb a flight of stairs, and there is the possibility of more serious health effects. (Tobacco is responsible for 7 million deaths per annum worldwide, according to the World Health Organization.)

There are plenty of other reasons to quit, not to mention: To save money, having healthy skin, for your kids, becoming more active, etc.

But if most smokers want to quit, have multiple reasons to quit, and realize just how dangerous cigarettes are to their health, what stops them from doing so?

The reason for that is clear. Nicotine addiction is deeply rooted in the subconscious mind. Stress, driving, mealtime, drinking (and the list goes on) all subconsciously cause cigarette cravings.

But what if your head had a way of "shutting off" the voice? Or at least reframe the subconscious thoughts to think about smoking negatively?

Well, this is the promise of hypnotherapy to quit smoking.

The smoker can begin to untangle and silence the web of subconscious thoughts that hold the addiction in place with the aid of a hypnotherapist or through self-hypnosis.

The Mental Trap: Why Can't You Stop Smoking

Because of physical and mental addiction, nicotine is such a hard habit to kick.

Physical addiction-which can cause withdrawal symptoms - serves as a roadblock to quitting.

Nicotine withdrawal causes:

- Aches and pains
- Sore throat
- Nausea
- Irritability
- Headache
- Mental sluggishness

But although the symptoms of nicotine withdrawal are painful, something is happening at a deeper level which makes it so difficult to quit smoking.

Mental addiction. Our subconscious emotions sustain the nicotine addiction. After dinner, or when you get behind the wheel, the subconscious causes the urge for a cigarette ... It's the subconscious mind that causes a pang when you're under stress.

This mental struggle also explains why most smoking cessation aids are ineffective, such as nicotine replacement therapy. Only physical cravings are eliminated by NRT – but those subconscious thoughts, those mental urges that tell us to reach for a cigarette are still very much in place.

But overcoming nicotine addiction requires smokers to fight the head-on mental battle. Thanks to top-down processing, the battle rages in your subconscious.

What is processed by top-down? Suppose a smoker who wants to quit has a major presentation at work. She is definitely feeling stressed out. The need for a cigarette might then be triggered by stress. But from where does this trigger originate?

Top-down processing may be effective in understanding the phenomenon.

In a nutshell, all the sensory information we obtain is sent to the brain - smell, touch, sights, feelings. The raw sensory data is transferred to the brain, where it produces a conscious perception. The brain then shapes feelings and emotions and provides a response.

In other words, the mind receives the signal of stress, thinks about what is going on and then generates a response that is focused on those thoughts.

It is the process that makes it so difficult to stop smoking.

Subconscious thoughts influence our top-down responses. You may associate smoking as a stress reliever, for example, and therefore your normal response to stress might be to light up.

The trick to stopping smoking is to gain top-down control- suppressing the unconscious reinforcement response that holds the addiction in place.

How Hypnosis Can Help You Quit:

One theory of why hypnosis works for addiction to nicotine: It allows us the opportunity to reframe our top-down thoughts.

Once you encounter stimuli that can induce craving, the mind has connections already in place that affect the response. You feel stressed out. The stress triggers smoking thoughts as a stress reliever. And you have responded.

However, hypnosis helps you get to a state of mind where you change the mechanisms of negative thinking.

How? Well, you follow relaxation and breathing strategies during hypnosis to achieve a trance-like state. This state of mind is similar to daydreaming; you are conscious, but the mind is detached at the same time.

Your mind is much more open to suggestions in the trance-state. It's disconnected from the critical, conscious mind – the part of the mind that is actively trying to remain a smoker.

Hence, a hypnotherapist will give you more constructive ideas to use. In other words, you are setting up roadblocks for the automatic, top-down mechanisms that keep the addiction in place. And when you experience a smoking trigger, the mind does not react automatically – it slows down to "listen" to this new information that you've received.

Reframing Your Subconscious Thoughts

Our subconscious thoughts are powerful and shape our perceptions. And when our subconscious tells us that this will work, we send the information back through top-down processing.

Hypnosis works in a similar fashion. We bring fresh, more detailed knowledge about smoking to our minds.

Hypnotic suggestions – those offered while in the state of trance – may concentrate on how habits are automatic reactions to thoughts, and how we have full control over our thoughts. Or you might be given ideas that rethink the smell of cigarette smoke, that is, it smells like burning plastic.

Additionally, one of the most common hypnosis techniques for smoking cessation is called the Spiegel's Method. One of the first psychiatrists to popularize therapeutic hypnotherapy, Herbert Spiegel was the author of "Trance and Treatment: Clinical Uses of

Hypnosis."

Spiegel would provide three repeated suggestions in a hypnosis script during the sessions including:

- Smoking is poison
- You should love your body and protect it
- You need your body to live

Spiegel's method did not focus on talking about stopping smoking. Actually, he theorized that making patients concentrate on respecting the body was key to changing destructive behavior.

Research Review: Stop Smoking with Hypnosis

We have touched on the hypnosis theory for stopping smoking. However, we haven't answered your question yet: Will hypnosis actually help you stop smoking?

The quick response is yes. Hypnosis has been found by some compelling studies to be an efficient tool to help you quit – with quit rates that easily beat more conventional methods.

Yet, like with any smoking cessation program, the consensus seems to be that you have to want the results. The best option is not hypnotherapy if:

- You feel like you should stop, but you don't really want to.
- You aren't ready to quit.
- You want to quit for someone else.

However, if you're ready, hypnosis can be an effective tool. A classic research on hypnosis explored the use of hypnotherapy across a variety of conditions. The study found that hypnotherapy needs an average of just six sessions of hypnotherapy to create a long-lasting improvement, whereas psychoanalysis takes 600.

It was seen that hypnosis was highly effective after six sessions 93% of participants, while the psychoanalysis group had a recovery rate of just 38%.

Several other studies have found evidence that hypnosis is a useful therapy for smoking cessation.

A scientific study at the American College of Chest Physicians conducted in 2007 compared hypnosis to nicotine replacement therapy. At 26 weeks, 50% of patients enrolled in the hypnotherapy group were still non-smokers, compared to only 15.78% in the nicotine replacement group. Patients of NRT and hypnotherapy have had a success rate of 50% at 26 weeks.

A study published in Psychological Reports in 1994 examined the effectiveness of hypnotherapy in combination with aversion therapy. In the research, a cessation program was undertaken by 93 male and 93 female participants, incorporating both approaches. About 90% of both groups abstained from smoking after three months.

A research published in the International Journal of Clinical and Experimental Hypnosis in 2001 examined the effectiveness of hypnosis and a quick smoking cessation protocol. The results: After

6 months, 39 of the 43 smokers who received treatment remained non-smokers.

A comprehensive meta-analysis reviewed more than 600 studies that examined various approaches for smoking cessation. The study has included more than 70,000 smokers. The study finds some convincing findings on hypnosis in general:

- Hypnosis was deemed two times more effective than self-help techniques, like quitting cold turkey or reading self-help books.

- Hypnosis was twice as effective as the nicotine gum replacement therapy

- Hypnosis was three times more effective than treatments by physicians involving more than counselling.

Are you ready to live a smoke-free life? Want to use hypnosis as an alternative for the therapy? You have many ways to use hypnosis to stop your cravings for smoking, all of which will help you curb your habit. The most popular of the three include:

- Private Hypnotherapy Sessions – You talk to a professional hypnotherapist directly. The hypnotherapist will ask you about your condition during a one-on-one session, which occurs over the phone, and then lead you through a hypnosis session.

- Recorded Sessions – Guided hypnosis sessions, typically available on a CD or as MP3s, offer a similar experience to private sessions. The main difference is the session is driven by a recording. You listen to the recording, following the steps to enter hypnosis.

- Self-hypnosis-Self-hypnosis appears to play a significant role in prevention of smoking. If you began with a private session, for example, you will possibly continue the therapy with self-hypnosis at home. In self-hypnosis, to enter the trance state, you undergo a hypnotic induction and then read from a hypnosis script to make suggestions to yourself. A quit smoking hypnosis script can also help.

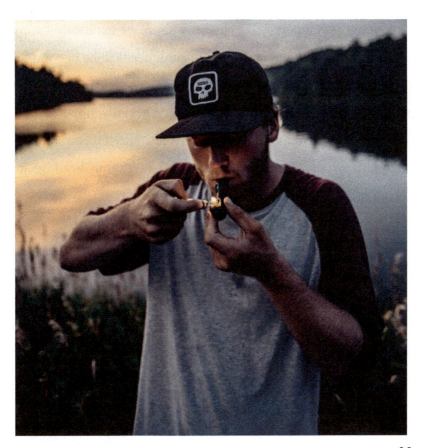

CHAPTER 3
IMPROVE YOUR STATE OF MIND AND FORM A HEALTHY MINDSET

When most people seek to become healthy, they just concentrate on physical features. They change their eating habits and follow a fitness routine. All truly great improvements to make, but the mental health of one is what sometimes gets ignored. When you want to be genuinely happy in life, both your physical and mental health needs to be in good form. If you are in a positive state of mind, you would be in a much better place to work in your daily life. It is especially important to be optimistic when you are facing challenges. Staying committed to a safe, active lifestyle is hard if you can't hold your head up in an upbeat space.

Here are ten tips that could just help you stay sunny and positive:

1. Accept Yourself for Who You Are.

    This one is huge. A lot of people struggle with self-esteem and self-worth every day. We're bombarded with images all day long and running comments telling us how we are "supposed" to look and act. If you continually compare yourself to others it can be difficult to find value. Striving for changes is necessary, but you must also note that you can only do it for you, not for anyone else. You are you and that is pretty awesome.

You are never going to look like anyone else. What you'll ever look like is a better you. In this world nothing is more important than doing the best you can.

2. Eat Healthy.

This is obvious because it is true. If you eat nothing but processed foods, nutritionally void, you will be doing yourself a disservice. When you eat healthy, fresh, whole foods, your body will function better and so will your brain. The processed foods contain chemicals that have a detrimental effect on your brain. When you are always feeling nervous or stressed out, consider cutting out caffeine and foods containing significant quantities of salt and sugar.

Check out BodyRock Meal Plan for some very nice meal ideas that will keep your body and mind healthy! This plan contains more than just a meal planner, a diet guide AND a recipe book with over 70 offers!

3. Surround Yourself with Positive People.

Being around positive people, and expressing your aspirations and dreams, will boost your well-being. Make time to see friends and relatives. Take time to laugh. Have fun together. These people who love you can make you feel confidence and joy. It is

so important to be appreciated for who you are.

If you have relationships that don't make you feel this way in your life, it may be time to re-examine whether they are worth keeping or not.

4. Appreciate the Little Things.

We are so busy that we can fail to consider the little stuff. Slow down, put all your electronics away. Breathe, then go for a walk. Take note of all you see. Take it in. Meditate. Kiss a dog. Doing stuff like this a couple of times a week helps to keep you grounded and aware of the things that really matter in life.

5. Find a Hobby.

Hobbies build skills and knowledge that will give you a sense of purpose in life. You just can't be about your workouts and job. Choose what pleases you. Your favorite hobbies will probably change over time but this is only a sign of progress. It's nice to have fun activities to look forward to!

6. Give Back to Others.

Some of the most important things you can do for your mental health is to do something nice for someone. When you feel like you've lost contact with any of the people that you care for, reach out to them and do something sweet. Doing something for someone else is only because one of the most blissful things you can do, and without the expectation of a return. The other person should not even be someone who you know. Are you stopping in the morning to get coffee when you're going to work? Pay for the person right behind you. You've done something nice to feel good about AND you have put an optimistic spin right off the bat on their day. Who knows, maybe they will be encourage to do the same. If this world needs one thing, it is more compassion.

7. Talk About Your Feelings.

Keeping your feelings locked inside is not good. You may not want to burden anyone else with your issues, but sharing them will help you work through your them. When you don't want to talk it out, consider writing in a journal. Not only would you have shared the feelings, but you can also go back and look at what you've written and understand yourself better.

8. Review Your Life Regularly.

Time stops for no one. The older we get, the easier it seems to fly. If you have a list of goals that you would like to achieve, don't forget to pause, check-in with yourself and track your progress. Sit down every few months, and look frankly at what you're doing in life. You can monitor your success and mark places that you want to develop.

9. Focus on What You Can Control.

Not everything will go as planned. And that is fine. Worrying about things you can't control would only stress you out. See what you will be in charge of. If this task always appears to be too large, split it up into smaller tasks. There'll always be something that you can't control in life. Identify it, and let go of it.

10. Use Failure to Promote Success.

If you get super bummed out after a failing, try to learn from it.

You may want to give up, but there is a lesson each time we struggle that will help us grow. Learn from these errors, and do the next time around better. When you allow yourself to wallow in failure, you will be convinced you can't. But you actually can. How do you maintain a healthy mindset?

10 WAYS TO PROMOTE A HEALTHY MINDSET

Being healthy is not about eating well and exercising, mental health also plays a major role in your overall well-being, but many of us fail to check-in and make time for a balanced mentality to practice. Around 1 in 4 Australians experience some form of mental illness, while others may experience occasional feelings of stress, lack of confidence or frustrated feelings.

There are a variety of different things you can do to cultivate a healthier attitude, from running to meditating, we share ten things you can do to encourage a healthy mindset and to support your best feeling.

1. **Eat well**

Research supports a diet of highly processed foods, with little nutrients, not only impacts the body but also the mind. Healthy nutrition from the inside out makes you feel good.

2. **Surround yourself with optimistic people**

Take the time to communicate with friends and family and the people around you. You'll feel happier and more comfortable by surrounding yourself with positive people. Many of us are running busy schedules, but it's important to make time to have fun and socialize.

3. **Take time to practice gratitude**.

It can be easy to forget to reflect for a minute or so and to think about the things you are thankful for in your life. Something as easy as having a cup of tea without technology, or meditation can go a long way in feeling happier and encouraging peace of mind.

4. **Avoid self-comparison**

For many people, comparison can take its toll resulting in a lower self-esteem or a lower sense of self-worth. Take comfort in the fact that nothing is the same and try to make time every now and then to disconnect from social media platforms.

5. **Find a hobby**

A balance between study and work and time spent doing things that make you happy will make a major difference to a healthy mindset. Do something new or take a lesson to make you feel fulfilled.

6. **Giving back**

Giving back to the community can help create meaningful connections with those around you, but it can also make your mentality stronger. Throughout the day, volunteer within your community or show small acts of kindness to those around you, and you'll feel better and happier.

7. **Talk about your feelings**.

It's important to share how we feel with people who are close to us. When you don't feel confident expressing your feelings with others, a personal journal will also help you to express what you experience.

8. Reflect

Making time to reflect is a powerful thing. Make time to reflect on the past day or week and talk about how you fixed problems and how it felt. Reflection is a perfect way to stick to yourself, learn and maintain a fresh mind.

9. Exercise

Many studies support the belief that exercise is very important in improving mental health. According to Knapen et. Al. (2014) exercise can boost body image, quality of life, resilience, and can also help in mild to moderate depression circumstances.

10. Use failure to encourage success.

Failure can be the foundation of personal development and growth. Only remember to pick yourself up again and try again!

CHAPTER 4
REDUCE ADDICTION-CAUSED ANXIETY AND STRESS

Stress and Anxiety

What are stress and anxiety?

Most people sometimes experience stress and anxiety. Stress is any demand that's put on your brain or body. People may report feeling stressed when they are put upon several competing demands. One event that makes you feel nervous or frustrated may activate the feeling of being stressed. Anxiety is a feeling of fear, anxiety or uneasiness. It can be a response to stress, or it can occur in individuals who cannot identify major stressors in their lives.

Stress and anxiety don't always get worse. They will help you overcome a problem or a dangerous situation in the short term. Symptoms of everyday stress and anxiety include stressing about finding a job, feeling nervous before a major exam, or being uncomfortable in certain social situations. If we haven't felt any anxiety, we might not be motivated to do things we need to do (for example, studying for that tough exam!).

Nonetheless, if stress and anxiety begin to interfere with your daily life, this can signify a more serious problem. If you avoid circumstances because of unreasonable fears, constantly worrying, or experience extreme anxiety about a traumatic incident weeks after it has occurred, it might be time to seek assistance.

What do Stress and Anxiety Feel Like?

Stress and anxiety can cause physical as well as psychological symptoms. People experience different anxiety and stress differently. Physical symptoms common to all include:

- headache
- rapid breathing
- fast heartbeat
- stomachache
- muscle tension
- sweating
- shaking
- change in appetite
- fatigue
- trouble sleeping
- diarrhea
- dizziness

- frequent urination

Anxiety and stress can also cause mental or emotional symptoms. Which may include:

- feelings of impending doom
- irrational anger
- restlessness
- panic or nervousness, especially in social settings
- difficulty concentrating

People who have long periods of stress and anxiety may experience negative health-related outcomes. These are more likely to develop high blood pressure, diabetes, heart disease,

and can also experience panic disorder and depression.

What causes anxiety and stress?

Stress and anxiety do come and go for most people. Typically, they happen after specific events in life, but then they go away.

Common causes

Common stressors include:

- having a friend or family member who is ill or injured
- death of a family member or friend
- moving
- starting a new school or job

- having an illness or injury
- getting married
- having a baby

Drugs and Medications

Drugs containing stimulants can make stress and anxiety symptoms worse. Daily use of caffeine, illicit drugs like cocaine and even alcohol can also aggravate the symptoms.

Prescription medications that can make the symptoms worse include:

- asthma inhalers
- thyroid medications
- diet pills

Stress and Anxiety-related Disorders

Stress and anxiety that occur regularly or seem out of proportion to the stressor may be indicators of an anxiety disorder. An estimated 40 million Americans live with an anxiety disorder of some kind.

People with these disorders can experience anxiety and stress on a daily basis and for prolonged periods of time. Such conditions may include:

- Generalized anxiety disorder (GAD) is a rising anxiety disorder characterized by uncontrollable worries. Often people are concerned about negative things that happen to them or to their loved ones and at other times they might not be able to find any source of concern.

- **Panic disorder is a condition that triggers panic attacks, which are moments of extreme anxiety followed by a pounding heart, fear of impending doom, and shortness of breath.**
- **Post-traumatic stress disorder (PTSD) is a condition causing hallucinations or anxiety arising from a traumatic encounter.**
- **Social phobia is a disorder that induces extreme anxiety sensations in conditions involving contact with others.**
- **Obsessive-compulsive disorder is a disease that induces repetitive thoughts and desire for certain ritual actions to be completed**

When to Seek Help

If you have thoughts of hurting yourself or others, then you can receive urgent medical assistance. Stress and anxiety are treatable disorders, and they can improve with many tools, techniques and therapies. When you can't contain your thoughts, and stress affects your daily life, speak to your primary care provider about ways to relieve stress and anxiety.

Techniques to Manage Stress and Anxiety

From time to time, it is normal to experience stress and anxiety and there are methods that you can use to make them more manageable. Pay attention to how the body and mind react to circumstances that are stressful and cause anxiety. You'll be able to predict your response the next time a traumatic event happens and it will be less disruptive.

Managing daily stress and anxiety

Certain changes in lifestyle can help relieve stress and anxiety symptoms. Both methods can be used in conjunction with traditional anxiety therapies. Stress and anxiety managing strategies include:

- getting enough sleep
- getting regular exercise
- meditating
- eating a balanced, healthy diet
- limiting caffeine and alcohol consumption
- scheduling time for hobbies
- recognizing the factors that trigger your stress
- talking to a friend
- keeping a diary of your feelings
- practicing deep breathing

Be careful if you tend to use substances such as drugs or alcohol to deal with stress and anxiety. It can lead to severe drug abuse problems that can worsen stress and anxiety.

Seek medical assistance to deal with stress and anxiety

There are several ways to seek treatment for anxiety and stress. If you feel you cannot cope with stress and anxiety, your primary care provider can recommend you see a provider of mental health care. I may use psychotherapy, also known as talk therapy, to help you work through your anxiety and stress. Your therapist can also teach you relaxation methods that will help you deal with stress.

A common and effective approach for managing anxiety is cognitive behavioral therapy (CBT). This form of therapy helps you to identify and change anxious thoughts and behaviors into more optimistic ones.

Exposure therapy and systemic desensitization can be beneficial for phobias treatment. We involve introducing you slowly to anxiety-provoking triggers to better control your feeling of fear.

Medications

The primary care provider can also prescribe medicine to help treat an anxiety condition that has been diagnosed. This may include selective serotonin reuptake inhibitors (SSRIs) such as paroxetine (Paxil) or sertraline (Zoloft). Providers often use anti-anxiety medications (benzodiazepines), such as or lorazepam (Ativan), or diazepam (Valium). Still, these methods are typically used on a short-term basis because of the risk of addiction.

What is the long-term outlook for stress and anxiety?

Stress and anxiety can be unpleasant to deal with. When untreated for long periods, they can also have detrimental effects on your physical health. While there is likely to be some amount of stress and anxiety in life and should not be cause for concern, it is important to understand when the stress in your life is having negative consequences. If you feel your stress and anxiety becomes unmanageable, look for professional assistance or ask others to help you find the support you need.

Does Stress Cause Addiction?

Historically, addiction was believed to result from consumption of an "addictive" substance, such as heroin or alcohol. Such substances were believed to have almost magical powers, making the user helpless over their use, irrespective of context and situations such as the user's stress. The DSM-IV definition of substance dependence focused on these substances' physiological effects and tolerance and withdrawal mechanisms as essential to addiction.

Since the 1970s, however, work has started to emerge that paints a different image of stress and dependency. Not only has it become clear that certain people who take "addictive" substances are not becoming addicted, but also that seemingly normal habits, not involving ingesting substances, have started to be recognized as addictive, including problem gambling, food addiction, computer addiction, shopping addiction, and even sex addiction. The set and setting and other contextual issues, such as the stress felt by the person taking the addictive substance or engaging in addictive behavior, are increasingly recognized as affecting whether or not people become addicted. The more recent findings are reflected in the DSM-V.

How Addiction is Used to Deal with Stress

Addiction often seems to be an attempt to deal with stress in a way that doesn't work quite well for the individual. While the drug or behavior you become addicted to can provide some temporary relief from stress, that relief is short-lived, so you need more to continue coping with stress. Because many addictions carry with them additional stress, such as the effects of withdrawal experienced when a drug wears off, even more of the addictive substance or activity is required to cope with the additional stress.

It is obvious from this viewpoint that some people are more vulnerable to addictions than others, simply because of the amount of tension they have in their lives. For example, there is now a well-established correlation between childhood violence, whether physical, emotional or sexual abuse and the subsequent development of substance and behavioral addictions. Childhood abuse is particularly traumatic to the child, but it tends to trigger issues as the child matures as an adult, with subsequent relationship and self-esteem issues. Not everyone who has been abused as a child develops an addiction and not everyone with addiction in childhood has been abused.

The vulnerability of child abuse survivors to subsequent addiction is a direct indication of the correlation between stress and addiction.

Although stress doesn't cause addiction on its own — many people are under stress and do not become an alcoholic — it plays a major role for others. Recognition of the role of stress in the development of addiction and the importance of stress management in preventing and overcoming addiction is important in helping people to avoid the pain that addiction can bring to both addicts and their loved ones. It is never too early to teach young people and children good stress management skills, so they are less inclined to become addicted.

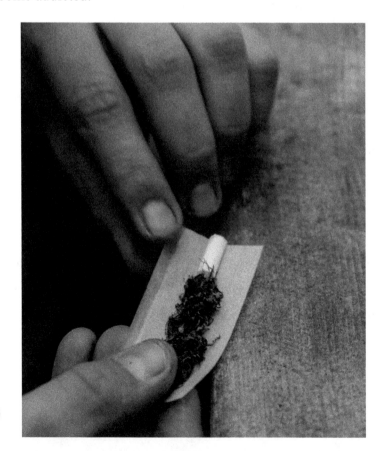

HOW DEPRESSION, ANXIETY AND ADDICTION GO TOGETHER AND WHY IT MATTERS

The most surprising statistic I have read about mental health is as follows: more than 50 percent of people in America will experience a mental disorder at some stage in their lives. This data comes from a report conducted by Harvard Medical School and the National Mental Health Institute (NIMH).

Take a moment to allow this to sink in. Then ask yourself, how much do we know about those circumstances that affect most of us in our lives at some point? Mental health issues aren't "side problems" they affect millions of Americans every day.

This year's National Depression Screening Day is on October 8, and the World Mental Health Day follows on October 10. Now is the perfect time to focus on depression and anxiety, two interrelated conditions of mental and emotional health which often precipitate addiction.

Depression and Anxiety by the Numbers

More than 8.3 million American adults have depression and anxiety, according to a 2017 report released in the journal Psychiatric Services. Plus, the 2016 Surgeon General's addiction report notes that in 2015, more than 27 million people abused drugs and more than 66 million abused alcohol.

Depression, anxiety, and addiction are growing, and they are all intertwined. However, let's describe those words before we think about why depression and anxiety contribute to drug addiction.

Defining Anxiety and Depression

Depression and anxiety are traditional textbook definitions which describe symptoms, not causes.

If you google "depression," you'll get this: "A mental health disorder characterized by persistently depressed mood." If you search for "anxiety," you'll find this: "A mental health disorder characterized by feelings of worry, anxiety, or fear." These definitions are accurate, but they're not exactly illuminating. The root causes aren't revealed.

We like to define depression as "anger turned inward." It's only three words in length, but it gets right to the heart of the matter. Depression is anger you weren't allowed to feel or express yourself. Though depression manifests in the form of numb apathy or sadness, it begins as anger.

Similarly, we define anxiety as "emotional energy bouncing back and forth, caught between the inner walls." Anxiety is the feeling you get when you refuse to feel your "off-limits," such as anger and hurt.

We teach a structure that clarifies the relationship between anxiety, depression, and addiction. It's called the "Anger-Hurt-Loving" model, and it points the path to recovery.

Depression, Anxiety, and Addiction

The Anger-Hurt-Loving model peels the curtain back and allows us to glimpse what usually drives addictive behaviors: untreated mental and emotional health problems. The model is also crucial to understanding anger and addiction.

Here's what it looks like

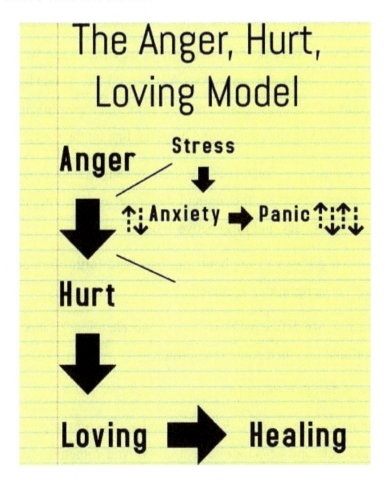

Here is an explanation of how it functions:

- There is an underlying hurt behind any feeling of wrath. When there's something we can't handle or what we need is absent, we get angry. Anyway, the reason we're angry is that it hurts a part of us.

- However, many of us were socialized not to feel our anger or express it, so we force it down and inward. The model's first diagonal line reflects how we cut off from the feeling of anger. Anger turned inward becomes depression.

- We've refused to feel our anger now, chances are we don't even want to feel our hurts. (Who would like to feel hurt? It hurts!) And we also cut off from that painful feeling experience, thus the second diagonal line on the model.

- Because we don't feel our hurt or anger, our emotional energy, that is, the up-and-down arrows in the model, bounces back and forth between our inner walls.

So, what do we call the bouncing back and forth of emotional energy? That's right; this is anxiety.

Likewise, we define panic as "anxiety acceleration." If anxiety is an emotional jog, then panic is a sprint.

How Addiction Plays In

And now we're anxious, depressed, and at the point of panic. We feel miserable and desperate to feel good. And sometimes the bar isn't even that high; we just feel so bad for a break! We want our feelings of anxiety, stress, and panic to be avoided, so we resort to substances. We use it not because we are bad, but because we feel bad.

Fortunately, there is a different option. Like you see in the picture, you step toward healing when you encourage yourself to feel your feelings rather than covering them up.

The best way to sum up the key message of the Anger-Hurt-Loving Model is this: When you apply love to the hurting parts of yourself, you recover.

You might think, Wait a minute, what about my medications? Don't they help me recover too?

The Role of Medications in Healing

While self-medication with illegal substances is dangerous, taking legally prescribed medications such as SSRIs for depression and anxiety can do a lot of good. Prescription drugs can help and stabilize people with mood disorders ... to some extent.

(Important clarification: we are not talking here about antipsychotic medications, since they are a separate class of medications with different protocols.)

Depression medicine can well be the right solution in the short term. But, in the long term, addressing the root causes is critical, not just alleviating the symptoms.

I do want to make people feel better. I want to provide crisis care. However, I want to provide people with the support they need to heal from depression and anxiety too.

Usually, I recommend people to maintain their current medications and dosages while they continue to resolve the underlying core issues. When they've been given enough time to meet with a doctor, they can determine if a lower dosage is needed. I

also see chronic mental health issues decreasing in severity-or even totally disappearing! – As people begin to show love to the part of themselves that hurt.

How to Treat Depression and Anxiety for Recovery

What is really behind your anxiety, mood swings, your depression? It's time to find out. It's time to treat the mental health problems instead of just medicating them and hope they're going to go away.

As you now know, lasting recovery from substance abuse involves treating and repairing the underlying core issues that originally triggered depression and anxiety. So, give yourself the tools and encouragement to deal through the anger and hurt you've been keeping in place. This could well mean ambulatory treatment. Perhaps this means seeking inpatient depression treatment. Everyone is different, but nobody should have to do it alone.

If you're afraid to feel and afraid to try, don't be. In offering this love and care to yourself, you will find that you are far stronger than you know.

As speaker and author Anne Lamott wrote:

"Hope begins in the dark, the persistent belief that the dawn will come if you just show up and try to do the right thing. You wait, watch, and work: you do not give up."

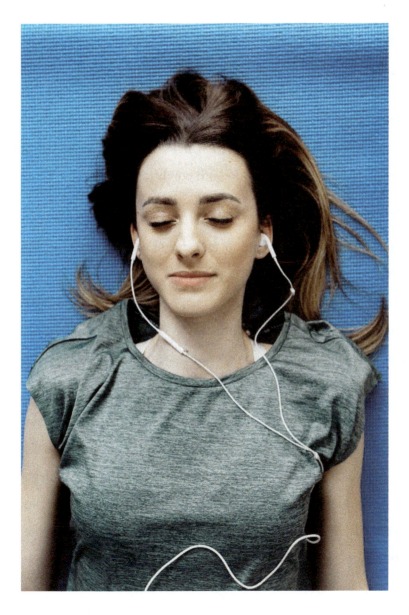

CHAPTER 5

ANXIETY DISORDERS AND DRUG ADDICTION

Approximately 18% of the U.S. population suffers from some form of anxiety disorder. Those who do are about two to three times more likely to have addiction problems than those who do not have anxiety. When a person has both substance disorder and mental health, this is known as dual diagnosis. Treatment can tackle both conditions.

Substance Abuse and Anxiety

Everyone experiences anxiety and stress. While most people may experience anxiety often in a fleeting way, the anxiety may be unrelated to some specific situation for a person with an anxiety disorder. And, it could be completely out of proportion to the actual situation. A severe anxiety problem affects your ability to function in your everyday life.

Some individuals with anxiety have a dual diagnosis, meaning they both have a mental condition, such as anxiety, and a substance abuse disorder. For these cases, it can be difficult to say which came first: the anxiety disorder or the substance abuse disorder. Some people with anxiety may use alcohol or drugs to self-medicate or better manage their symptoms.

Comorbidity is common with substance abuse and anxiety; this means people frequently face the 2 conditions together. Approximately 20 percent of those with anxiety or mood disorder have substance abuse problems, just as approximately 20 percent of those with a substance abuse problem have anxiety or mood disorder.

Risk Factors

While anxiety and the substance abuse are separate disorders, they carry common risk factors like:

- Genetic vulnerability. Genetic components can have some similarity that increases a person's susceptibility to developing both anxiety and addiction and disorders.

- Environmental triggers. Examples include abuse and trauma, which can also lead to anxiety as well as increased vulnerability to substance use.

- Involvement of similar brain regions. The functioning of the brain is also a common factor in both forms of disorder. For people with anxiety and other mental health conditions, main brain regions that respond to reward and stress and are affected by drugs may also show irregularities.

- Developmental stages. It is likely that teenage drug use can affect certain brain functions in a way that makes them more vulnerable to drug effects and contributes to anxiety disorders.

Symptoms

There are several types of anxiety disorders, with symptoms varying slightly. The generalized anxiety disorder (GAD) symptoms include:

- An inability to concentrate.
- Being irritable.
- Tense muscles.
- Being unable to control worrying.
- Feeling restless or on edge.
- Getting tired easily.
- Problems getting to sleep, feeling rested, or staying asleep.

Panic disorder includes symptoms such as:

- Worries and fears of another attack occurring.
- Sudden attacks of fear.
- Avoiding places in which attacks have occurred.
- Loss of control over the feelings of fear.

People with social anxiety have symptoms such as:

- Getting sick physically when having to interact with others.
- Difficulty interacting with others.
- Avoiding people as much as possible.

- Blushing, sweating, or having issues speaking when others are around.
- Being very worried about judgment by others.
- Having difficulty making and keeping friends.

A variety of symptoms are associated with addiction to alcohol and drugs. An individual may be diagnosed with a substance abuse disorder if they display at least 2 of these symptoms at any point in the past twelve months:

- Taking more of the drug than they expected.
- Continued usage despite being mindful of the legal ramifications.
- Continued use, despite knowledge of the adverse effects of the medication (for instance, emotional health or deteriorating medical).
- Strong craving for the substance of abuse.
- Inability to cut back on using drugs or alcohol.
- Failure to do what you are supposed to do at school, at home, or at work, and failure to fulfil your obligations due to alcohol or drugs.
- Alcohol or drugs take on greater significance than previous interests or hobbies.
- Doing irresponsible things, like driving while on drugs or

alcohol.

- Alcohol and drugs typically eat up your time. Whether you're using drugs and alcohol, or you're trying to get over it, or you're trying to get more alcohol and drugs.

- Increased tolerance of the alcoholic or drug substance to where more is required to develop the desired feelings. Stopping use or cutting back triggers withdrawal symptoms.

ANXIETY AFTER DRUG USE

Sometimes during or after drug use, a person can experience panic attacks or general anxiety. The Mental Disorders Diagnostic and Statistical Manual explain that if the anxiety occurs during or soon after intoxication and leads to impairment in social or occupational functioning, a person may be diagnosed with a substance-induced anxiety disorder.

Drugs that may cause anxiety disorder with the substance include alcohol, PCP (phencyclidine), inhalants, stimulants, and hallucinogens.

Other drugs can cause anxiety when the person starts taking the medications and withdrawal experiences. Usually, this form of anxiety occurs with drugs that inhibit the central nervous system and relieve anxiety, including benzodiazepines, opioids, and alcohol.

Symptoms of drug-induced anxiety from withdrawal can include:

- Shaking.
- Elevated blood pressure.
- Hyperactivity.
- Agitation.

For some people, marijuana reduces anxiety. Others may actually experience increased anxiety, though, particularly when they use marijuana at higher doses. Many individuals, genetic, and environmental factors can lead to marijuana-induced anxiety. Women, those who rarely use marijuana and those with pre-existing anxiety disorders are more vulnerable to marijuana-induced anxiety than others.

Treatment

When a person has both a mental illness such as anxiety and a substance use disorder, all conditions must be treated. A person who only completes drug recovery and does not receive anxiety treatment is more likely to experience medical complications, suicide or early death.

In addition to living a healthy lifestyle, which requires exercise, a healthy diet, and proper nutrition, both conditions may be treated with medication. But if treatment combines the drugs with therapy, the person would likely have a better outcome.

Medications

Anxiety disorders are also treated with antidepressants medication. Commonly used antidepressants include both SNRIs (selective norepinephrine inhibitors) and SSRIs (selective serotonin reuptake inhibitors). Some people may be prescribed benzodiazepines for short-term anxiety control which include drugs such as Valium and Xanax.

The risk of addiction, however, makes such drugs less than ideal for people with history of drug abuse.

Alcoholism can be treated with disulfiram (Antabuse) and acamprosate (Campral). These drugs produce an unpleasant reaction when one drinks and, respectively, decreases withdrawal symptoms. Naltrexone, a drug used to treat opioid addiction, can also work in the treatment of alcohol addiction.

For people with opioid dependence, there are many medication-assisted drugs for recovery. As in treatment for alcohol dependence, naltrexone can be used to block some of the opioid's rewarding effects, thus discouraging continued use.

Other medicines, such as buprenorphine and methadone, tend to stop the cravings and relapse of opioid-related symptoms, making them helpful during detox and maintenance therapy.

Therapies

Numerous therapies help treat addiction and anxiety. The most popular addiction treatments are:

- Cognitive behavioral therapy, or CBT, helps change a person's mindset about drugs and using strategies to cope with the stress. CBT also helps a person learn how to identify drug addiction triggers and how to prevent or cope with these triggers.
- Motivational interviewing. This approach increases the ability of an individual to get involved in the process of

change. Among those who need addiction treatment, ambivalence can be found, particularly if a court or legal program has ordered the treatment program. Instead of ignoring this ambivalence, motivational interviewing identifies that and tries to help people work through it.

- Contingency management. This uses rewards, such as vouchers or gift cards for negative drug screens to help people stay engaged in treatment.
- Matrix Model.
- This method is most widely used to treat stimulants addiction to. The program utilizes urine drug screens, 12-step groups, individual therapy, family therapy, and drug education.
- Exposure therapy. This form of CBT therapy slowly introduces the person to a situation or an object that makes them very anxious. At each stage of the process, they are taught to manage the anxiety.
- Relaxation training. Relaxation training is often a part of exposure therapy and CBT. Mindfulness is also integrated and can include meditation or the visualization of relaxing scenes. Furthermore, the training involves self-soothing methods, such as using oils and scents. Physical relaxation involves learning to relax muscles, doing activities such as yoga, and breathing calmly.
- Breathing training. Breathing training involves learning to

breathe deeply, from the diaphragm, holding the breath, and exhaling gradually, all of which will usually help a person feel less anxious.

Anxiety disorders are most often treated with CBT. For disorders such as panic disorders or social anxiety, the number of patients receive 12 to 16 sessions over a span of 3 to 4 months. The anxiety disorders, however, appear to be chronic. Recurrence is common even after treatment. Some people require a longer recovery plan which can last up to 50 sessions or more than a year.

Recovery Programs

Recovery programs are widely available. Forms of treatment include:

- Inpatient treatment. An inpatient program will offer 24/7 medical, supervision, and social support to help a person stop using drugs while also learning how to manage their anxiety.

- Outpatient treatment. For some people, outpatient treatment programs can be an option to receive anxiety and addiction treatment. Outpatient treatment programs vary in how often a person is attending treatment. Most outpatient programs may meet at a time for only one day or 2 per week, for 2 to 3 hours. Some programs, however, include an intensive outpatient program, or IOP, which normally meets for 2-3 days a week, generally 3-4 hours a day. Other treatment programs provide what is known as partial hospitalization, or PHP, which typically meets 4-6 hours a day, from five to seven days a week.

Often, such programs are the initial stage of treatment. Other times, people will attend PHP or IOP as a step away from a more serious type of treatment, such as hospital treatment. Service intensity is contingent upon individual needs.

Other types of programs that may be incorporated into outpatient or inpatient programs or used as follow-up care to treatment include:

- Twelve-step programs. Such programs are usually an aftercare form for someone who has been through a course of outpatient and/or inpatient treatment. However,

- some people are using them as their main source of recovery. These groups are vital to ongoing sobriety and support.

- Support groups. This can be run by a therapist or other individuals who have been dealing with or have dealt with anxiety. These groups are useful in finding other people in the same situation as you, and in learning how to handle their own anxiety.

HOW TO STOP SMOKING AND STAY CALM IN THE PROCESS

The coronavirus (COVID-19) pandemic has changed the way we all live our lives. A new world of practices of self-isolation and social distancing will likely remain in place for some time to slow the spread of the virus.

This may leave you feeling more worried, anxious, and stressed because you lack the social interaction that makes you feel connected and optimistic.

You may feel overwhelmed by additional concerns about your health, the health of your family and your job. Such feelings can affect anyone and are difficult to deal with, and can make it particularly difficult to stop smoking at this time.

Good Thinking and Stop Smoking London have teamed up with that in mind to give smokers some tips on how to quit – and how to remain calm in the process.

Understand the Role Anxiety Plays in Smoking

We know it can be difficult to quit smoking, and it can feel especially difficult at this time. Some of you may turn to cigarettes in the belief that smoking is going to help to relieve stress and anxiety – but it does not! Smoking relieves symptoms of nicotine withdrawal such as irritability and low mood-tricking you into thinking that it helps with stress. It has been shown that people who stop smoking have less depression, anxiety, and stress, plus improved mood compared to those who keep smoking.

1. **Use deep breathing and meditation to help reduce stress and anxiety**.

Using proven guided meditation and visualization methods is a great way to feel calmer when you stop smoking. Not only does this make you better, but it will also help you make certain healthier lifestyle choices.

2. Make a quit plan

You can move forward confidently with your stop-smoking journey by giving yourself time to prepare. Get support and use a stop smoking medication, such as a patch and another nicotine product, or some prescription medications, to greatly increase your chances of stopping successfully.

It also helps prepare yourself for those situations and feelings that may cause you to smoke.

3. Get lots of sleep

Sleep disturbances are a common side effects of nicotine withdrawal. Lack of sleep will make it feel so much harder like quitting smoking. So, getting on top of any sleep problems that you may encounter quickly is especially important.

4. Exercise daily

Scheduling outdoor exercise as often as you wish is recommended and is good for you – as long as you meet the recommendations for social distance.

Exercising 30 minutes a day is a perfect self-help practice to get the endorphins flowing and improve strength. When you stop smoking, you can find that you have less coughing and shortness of breath as your lungs recover, which makes exercise easier. It will also improve your mood by being more involved, relieving stress and help you to sleep better.

5. Don't do it by yourself, ask for help

The final tip is to see how you feel about these feelings and be compassionate. It may help you to speak about them with your family and friends using phone or video calls. Online communities are also there to help you stop smoking.

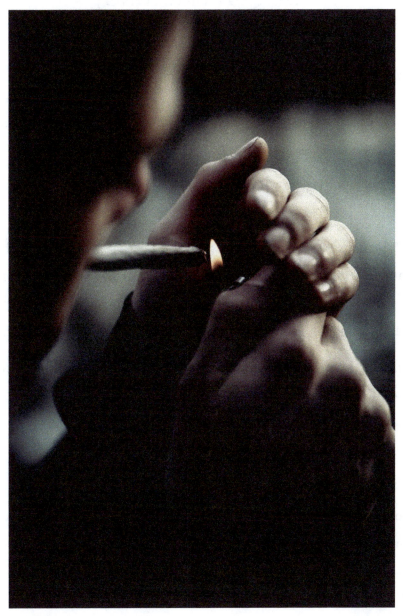

CHAPTER 6
WAYS TO RELIEVE INSOMNIA WHEN YOU QUIT SMOKING

New ex-smokers during the process of smoking cessation will sleep more than normal. This can leave you feeling confused and lethargic as your body responds to the loss of multiple doses of nicotine and other chemicals during the day.

If this describes how you feel, do not fight off the need for extra sleep.

Take naps when you can, and get to bed earlier than usual. With a little rest, the body's going to bounce back. On the opposite side of the spectrum are the ex-smokers who have trouble getting to sleep at all. Insomnia is a common symptom of withdrawal from nicotine.

If you experience insomnia in the first few weeks after you stopped smoking, try some of these natural remedies to relieve your uneasiness.

1. **Cut Your Caffeine Intake in Half**

Smokers metabolize caffeine much more easily than non-smokers do. Smokers must also drink more caffeine to achieve the same effects as non-smokers.

If you stop smoking without lowering the consumption of caffeine, the body gradually becomes over-caffeinated, which can make you feel irritable and jittery. You may not be able to drink as much as you did as a smoker, though you don't need to cut caffeine out completely.

Start by reducing your consumption of caffeine by at least 50 percent This should give you the right amount of caffeine without feeling the symptoms of caffeine withdrawal or being over-caffeinated.

Gradually lower your intake of caffeine instead of going "cold turkey". Quitting caffeine altogether can lead to uncomfortable symptoms of withdrawal.

2. Take a Warm Bath

Light a few scented candles, use some fragrant bath salts and let go of the day's stress. A warm bath is a perfect way to relax and prepare the body and mind for sleep.

3. Schedule a Massage

Enlist your partner or other willing pair of hands to help work your muscles relieve the stress. Although a luxurious full body massage is fantastic, even 10 or 15 minutes spent on your shoulders, face, neck, and scalp can work wonders to help you unwind and get ready for a good night's sleep.

4. Drink a Cup of Tea

There are a variety of herbal teas specifically blended to help soothe and promote sleep. Take a look at the supermarket's tea section or visit your local health food store and ask for suggestions.

5. Listen to Soothing Music

Soothing, mellow music will help you to relax enough to drift off to sleep. Try to listen to a sound of waves lapping on the beach. Sounds of rain, thunder, and sounds of nature can be relaxing too. If you're listening to music on your phone or tablet while you fall asleep, make sure that it is set to automatically turn off.

You don't want to get up and do it yourself, because that's defeating the object.

6. Create a Digital Curfew

Using electronic equipment before bedtime will make it more difficult for you to fall and stay asleep. That is because the artificial blue light produced by devices such as smartphones, tablets and laptops suppresses melatonin production, the sleep-regulating hormone.

Consider turning off your electronics one to two hours prior to going to bed. Try to incorporate wind-down practices such as reading (an actual written book, not one on your phone) or meditation instead of screen time, to get your body ready for a good night's rest.

7. Drink a Glass of Warm Milk

Warm milk improves your sleep because it is full of a sleep-inducing amino acid known as tryptophan. The neurotransmitter serotonin, which is then transformed into the hormone melatonin, is produced by the body using tryptophan.

Your brain has more tryptophan available when you consume a carbohydrate along with it. No wonder milk and cookies have long been a popular snack in bedtime.

Other foods that contain tryptophan include:

- Fish
- Cheese
- Eggs
- Seeds (including sunflower seeds)
- Nuts (such as cashews, almonds, pistachios, and hazelnuts)
- Soy products (such as tofu and soy sauce)
- Poultry (such as turkey and chicken)

L-tryptophan supplements are usually not recommended, because they were historically associated with syndrome of eosinophilia-myalgia. Food and drink containing L-tryptophan, of course, are better options.

8. Don't Drink Alcohol.

Although a drink or two may initially make it easier to fall asleep, alcohol avoidance is best. Alcohol suppresses rapid eye movement (REM) sleep, ensuring you won't feel relaxed in the morning, even if you sleep through the evening. Alcohol in your body can also interrupt your sleep and cause you to wake up repeatedly during the night

9. Get Some Exercise

If you can't sleep, try to get out a few hours before bed for a good long stroll. Just a 15-minute walk will help. However, timing is vital with this one. Try to stop intense exercise at least one hour before bedtime because it can make it harder to fall asleep.

10. Relaxation Methods

Try meditation and progressive muscle relaxation at the end of a busy day, to ease your mind and relax your muscles.

Lie down with your eyes closed, try these simple relaxation methods in bed. Start to tense and relax the muscles throughout your body as an alternative, starting with your feet and working your way up.

Then, move on to your mental thoughts. Recognize each when it comes to mind and then let it go. Let the mind float and drift, relieving worry and stress as it goes.

11. Don't Nap During the Day.

While finally getting some shut-eye may feel good, if it's during the day, don't do it. If you are struggling with insomnia, power naps aren't your friend. You'll pay for it when it is time for bed.

12. Start Your Day a little earlier.

Another effective strategy is to start your day a little earlier to help you change your internal clock. You can also use the extra time to meditate – a win, a win.

The physical withdrawal phase of smoking cessation is a temporary condition. Your sleep habits would quickly return to normal if you had no insomnia before you stopped smoking. If symptoms continue for the first month or so, arrange an appointment with your doctor to ensure that smoking cessation is responsible for how you feel.

CHAPTER 7
POSITIVE AFFIRMATIONS TO QUIT SMOKING

Fed up with smoking?

Are you ready to heal your nicotine addiction?

Here is a list of the best positive affirmations and quotes that will help you stop smoking so you can control your life more.

Best Affirmations If You Want to Stop Smoking

1. I have decided to stop smoking, and it feels good.
2. I love myself more. I say "no" to smoking and "yes" to life.
3. It's easy to quit smoking.
4. I gain nothing as a smoker.
5. As a non-smoker I have a lot to gain.
6. Choosing to be free of nicotine is a choice which I am glad to make.
7. I just breathe and let go, anytime I need a break.
8. I care about my body and let go of addictions which are unhealthy.

9. I hereby release any need to smoke with open arms and accept a smoke-free life.

10. Smoking is no real fun, that's why I would find it easy to quit.

11. This is the moment I choose freedom from smoking.

12. I prefer a daily breath of fresh air.

13. Because I know myself better every day, I know how to easily quit smoking.

14. Quitting smoking takes no power because I do not want to smoke.

15. I'm going to be free from smoking and do it happily.

16. I'll stop smoking easily.

17. My natural state is that of a non-smoker.

18. Knowing I have control over my life decisions, including smoking, is empowering.

19. I opt for good health.

20. I look to the future with excitement, as a non-smoker.

21. My life as a non-smoker would be healthier.

22. I look forward to living a cigarette-free life.

Best Stop Smoking If You've Already Quit

1. Each day I feel happy and better in every way.

2. I prefer a daily breath of fresh air.

3. Every day, my lungs feel better.

4. I live a smoke-free life now, and that feels fantastic.

5. I choose not to smoke, and that feels good.

6. I appreciate that new sense of freedom I have as a non-smoker.

7. As a non-smoker today, I am engaged in activities that support my well-being.

8. My body is nicotine-free, and feels good.

9. Now I can say "I don't smoke". That gives me an immense sense of pride.

10. I love my body deeply and respect it.

11. As a non-smoker, my self-image increases every day.

12. I move away from smoking, towards a new, healthier me every single day.

13. Each day, my breathing is improving.

14. Being smoke-free, I now feel complete ease in all situations.

15. It's easy to eliminate Nicotine from my life.

16. Today, I'm free to smoke, and I'm really happy about it.

17. My lungs are becoming healthy and clean.

18. As a non-smoker, I am calm and relaxed.

19. Being free from cigarettes feels amazing.

20. As a non-smoker, my life gets better every day in every way.

21. I am so grateful that I have opted to give up cigarettes for health and happiness.

22. I feel happy when I wake up with the choice I made to be smoke-free.

Affirmations to Stop Smoking Forever

1. I never want to smoke again.
2. I let go of the urge to smoke.
3. Smoking no longer serves me.
4. I have control over my life.
5. I'm delighted to be breathing fresh air.
6. My lungs are clean and healthy.
7. I let go of my smoking addiction.
8. I can quickly conquer my smoking addiction.
9. I'm ready to stop smoking.

Affirmations to Overcome Smoking Addiction

1. I am not an addict.
2. I take life into my hands.
3. I'm stronger than cigarettes.
4. I am not nicotine addict.
5. I am motivated to stop smoking.

6. My goal is to be healthy.

7. I don't enjoy smoking.

8. My lungs are nicotine-free.

Affirmations to Find Inner Peace

1. I'm peaceful, calm and focused.

2. I'm free from addiction.

3. I find peace through meditation or taking a walk.

4. I'm more comfortable in non-smoking environments.

5. I find happiness within myself.

6. I am feeling at peace with myself.

7. I'm feeling happy and at ease.

8. My breathing is slow and calm.

Affirmations to Release Stress and Anxiety

1. I am letting go of my worries.

2. I have absolutely nothing to worry about.

3. My anxiety is fading away gradually.

4. I release any stress-related thoughts I have.

5. I choose to focus on the good stuff.

6. I am a less anxious person every day.

7. I'm filled with peace and calm.

8. My stress is disappearing.

Affirmations to Create Healthy Habits

1. I am in control of my habits.
2. I make good choices.
3. I enjoy maintaining a healthy lifestyle.
4. I am creating the life of my dreams. One choice at a time.
5. I love nourishing my body.
6. I am happy when I exercise.
7. I enjoy eating healthy foods.
8. I am motivated to be a healthy and fit person.
9. I am grateful for my willpower.
10. I am proud of myself for my choices.

Quotes & Sayings to Help You Quit Smoking

- Take control of your life. Take control of your habits – Anonymous.
- Out of our weakness, our strength rises — Ralph Emerson Waldo.
- We become what we repeatedly do — Sean Covey.
- Consistency creates habit, and habits shape our lives.
- Cigarette smoking is like paying to shorten your life.
- Every time you light up a cigarette, you are saying your life

is not worth living.

- It is at your moments of decision that your destiny is shaped – Tony Robbins.
- Smoking is harmful to the brain, hateful to your nose, and dangerous to the lungs – King James.
- Your craving is TEMPORARY, but it will damage your lungs PERMANENTLY.
- The key to breaking any bad habit successfully is to love something greater than habit – MacGill Bryant.
- We form habits first, then they form us. Conquer your bad habits, or they will conquer you eventually – Anonymous.
- To quit smoking, you must first want to quit, but then you must also do the quitting –Goethe.
- If it seems impossible to stop smoking right now, it is exactly what you should start doing – Eleanor Roosevelt.
- You really get closer to staying smoke-free each time you decide to stop smoking – Henry Ford.
- You're never going to change your life until you change something that you do every day. Your everyday routine is the secret to your success – John C. Maxwell.

Six Ways to Give Your Mind A Break:

1. Stop worrying.

2. Forget the problems weighing you down.

3. Stop stressing.

4. Lighten up.

5. Forgive others.

6. Forgive yourself — Germany Kent.

CHAPTER 8
RELAX AND FALL ASLEEP EASILY EVERY NIGHT

It can be frustrating to not be able to fall asleep and feel the consequences the next day. People will learn to fall asleep more easily using easy, natural tips and tricks.

When someone is having trouble falling asleep, one solution is to take sleep-inducing medications. These medications, however, aren't an ideal long-term remedy.

Certain natural methods — such as providing a regular bedtime routine, avoiding screens before bedtime, doing gentle daytime exercise, reading before bedtime, and practicing other strategies of mindfulness — can help.

Different things work for different people, so take some time to find out what works for you.

This chapter looks at twenty-one natural methods that people can use to fall asleep quickly.

Twenty-one Ways to Fall Asleep Naturally

Having a consistent sleep pattern can help a person fall asleep faster.

Most people struggling with sleep lie in bed, worrying about how to fall asleep. Consider following the guidelines below when this happens. Many of them are adjustments in lifestyle for the long term, and some are short-term approaches to try straight away.

1. Create a consistent sleeping pattern

Going to bed every night at various times is a common occurrence for many. Such irregular sleeping patterns, however, may interfere with sleep because they disrupt the circadian rhythm of the body.

The circadian rhythm is a combination of behavioral, mental, and physical changes over a cycle of 24 hours. A primary role of circadian rhythm is to determine whether or not the body is ready to sleep.

A biological clock which releases hormones to induce sleep or wakefulness heavily influences this. Going to bed at the same time every night helps the body clock determine when to trigger sleep.

2. Keep the lights off.

Cues like light also affect the circadian rhythm, which helps tell the brain and body when it's night. Keeping the room as dark as possible before going to bed can help bring on to sleep.

3. Avoid napping during the day.

Taking naps during the daytime can also disrupt the circadian rhythm, particularly those which last longer than 2 hours.

One study discovered that college students who slept at least three times a week and those who slept for more than two hours each time had a lower quality of sleep than their peers who did not.

It is tempting to take a long nap after a poor night's sleep. Try to prevent this because it can adversely affect a healthy sleep cycle.

4. Get some exercise during the day.

Physical exercise affects the quality of the sleep positively.

One study that looked at 305 people above the age of 40 with sleeping problems found that exercise programs of moderate to high intensity contributed to changes in sleep quality. The study also found participants took their sleep medication less often when taking part in an exercise program.

It is still uncertain whether or not exercise is having an effect on sleep at various times of the day.

When you embark on an exercise routine, it can be hard to know where to start.

5. Avoid using your cell phone.

There is currently much debate as to whether the use of cell phones at bedtime affects sleep or not.

One research on college students found that there was a poorer sleep quality for those who scored high on a scale of problem phone use, such as addictive texting behavior.

Most of the latest research is in students and young people, and it is unknown whether these results apply to other age groups or not. Research also appears to concentrate on the issue of phone usage.

People who do not use their phone in this manner may not be as prone to sleep disturbances.

In this area, more work is required to understand the extent to which phone usage can affect sleep.

6. Read a book

Reading books can be calming and can help avoid habits of worrying thoughts that could interfere with a person's sleep. It is best to avoid books which may trigger strong emotional

responses.

7. Avoid caffeine

Caffeine acts as a stimulant. This increases wakefulness and can interfere with sleep patterns. It is also best to avoid caffeine for at least four hours before bedtime.

Caffeine intake at any time of the day may have a detrimental impact on the quality of the sleep in certain people. It may be better for some individuals to avoid caffeine altogether.

8. Try meditation or mindfulness

Mindfulness and meditation can help reduce anxiety, which also disrupts sleep. Using these techniques can help to calm an anxious mind, distract the person from busy thoughts and make it easier for them to fall asleep.

A research in older adults with sleeping problems discovered that meditation increased the quality of sleep compared to people who didn't practice meditation.

9. Try counting

A longstanding method of sleep induction is to gradually count down from 100. There are a lot of theories about why this may work, including boredom and distracting the individual from anxious thoughts.

10. Change your eating habits.

What an individual eats can have an impact on their sleep, particularly in the evening. Eating a large meal within one hour of going to bed, for example, can hinder a person's ability to sleep.

It can take at least two to three hours to digest a meal. Lying down during this time can cause feelings of nausea or discomfort in certain people and slow down the digestive process.

Best to allow enough time for the body to digest a meal before lying down. The exact time it takes can vary from one person to another.

11. Get the room temperature right

Being too cold or too hot will affect a person's ability to sleep.

The temperature at which people feel most relaxed varies, so experimenting with different temperatures is necessary.

The National Sleep Foundation suggests a 60–67 ° F (16–19oC) bedroom temperature to encourage sleep.

12. Try aromatherapy

Aromatherapy has long been used by individuals to promote relaxation and sleep.

Lavender oil is a popular choice to aid sleep. A research in 31 young adults discovered that the use of lavender oil before bed had a beneficial impact on the quality of the night's sleep. After waking up, the participants reported having more energy.

13. Find a comfortable position.

Sleeping in a comfortable position is necessary. Changing positions frequently can be disruptive, but finding the right position will make a major difference to the onset of sleep.

Most people find that the best position for a good night's sleep is to lie on their side.

14. Listen to music

Though this does not work for everybody, some people benefit from listening to music that relaxes them before going to bed.

The response of a person to the music will depend on their personal preferences. Music can be distracting at times, but can cause anxiety and sleeplessness.

15. Try breathing exercises

Breathing exercises are a relaxation technique which is very popular. Practicing deep breathing or doing different breathing exercises will help de-stress people and take away worrying thoughts from their mind. It can be a tool to get to sleep.

One common option is 4-7-8 breathing. This involves breathing in for four seconds, holding the breath for 7 seconds, and exhaling for eight seconds. This kind of deep, rhythmic breathing is relaxing and may encourage sleep.

16. Take a hot bath or shower

It can be soothing to take a bath or shower and help prepare the body for sleep. This can also help enhance the control of temperature before bedtime.

Cold and hot showers have different benefits. Hot showers will help make you sleep better.

17. Avoid reading e-books

Over the past few years, e-books have become more popular.

They have backlit screens which make them perfect for reading in a dark room before bed. This may have a detrimental effect on sleep, though.

One study provided a printed book and an e-book for young adults to read before bed. The researchers found the participants had taken longer to fall asleep when using the e-book.

We were also more alert in the evenings and less alert throughout the morning due to reading the printed text. These findings suggest that e-books may have a detrimental effect on sleep.

The study did involve only 12 participants. The researchers also used a study design which meant participants were reading both kinds of books. It is difficult to determine whether or not exposure to both reading conditions has biased the results.

There are few reliable studies in this area, and any firm conclusions need require further research.

1. **Take melatonin**

Melatonin is known as the sleep hormone, which is generated by the body in order to cause drowsiness and sleep in line with the body clock. People may also take it as a replacement to improve the ability to get to sleep.

2. **Use a comfortable bed.**

The National Sleep Foundation advises that people sleep on a comfortable mattress, and cozy, supportive pillows to get a good night's sleep. Investing in comfortable mattress may have a beneficial effect on the quality of the sleep.

3. **Avoid noisy environments, if possible.**

Noise can be distracting, preventing the onset of sleep and decreasing sleep quality.

A 2016 study found participants in a hospital setting had significantly worse sleep than at home. The study authors found this was mainly due to the increased noise level in the hospital.

4. **Avoid excessive alcohol consumption.**

Drinking copious amounts of alcohol before bed will adversely affect sleep. Alcohol is problematic because it can give rise to feelings of restlessness and nausea, which can disrupt the onset of sleep.

CHAPTER 9
DEEP SLEEP ALL NIGHT LONG

What is Deep Sleep and Why is it Important?

What to know about deep sleep?

You may have learned that between 7 and 9 hours of sleep is required for adults every night.

When you rest, the body moves through various stages of the sleep cycle. For example, deep sleep is the stage of sleep you need when you wake up in the morning to feel refreshed. Unlike rapid eye movement (REM), deep sleep is when the body and brain waves are slowing down.

It's hard to wake up from deep sleep, and you may still feel tired if you do.

What Are the Stages of Sleep?

Sleep is divided into two groups: REM and non-REM sleep. You start the night in non-REM sleep, followed by a short period of REM sleep. The cycle continues at about every 90 minutes during the night.

Deep sleep occurs in the final stage of non-REM sleep.

Non-REM sleep

Stage 1 of non-REM sleep lasts several minutes as you transition from being awake to sleeping.

During stage 1:

- Your body functions — like respiration, eye movements, and heartbeat — begin to slow down
- Your muscles relax with occasional twitches
- Your brain waves start slowing down from wakeful state

Stage two accounts for approximately 50% of the overall cycle of sleep. This is the stage of sleep you may fall into more than any other throughout the night.

During stage 2:

- Decline in core temperature
- Your body systems continue to relax and slow down
- Your eye movement stops
- Your brain waves are weak, but you do have a few short activity bursts

Stages 3 and 4 are when you experience deep sleep

During these stages:

- It's hard to awaken even with loud noises
- As your muscles relax, your heartbeat and breathing become their slowest

- Your brain waves become the slowest they will be while you are asleep

Deep sleep is also known as "slow-wave sleep" (SWS) or delta sleep.

The first deep sleep stage lasts from 45 to 90 minutes. During the first half of the night, it lasts for longer periods and gets shorter with each sleep cycle.

REM sleep

Stage 5, or the first stage of REM sleep, occurs after going through non-REM periods for around 90 minutes.

During this stage:

- Your eyes move rapidly from side to side
- You experience a dream as your brain activity progresses to a more awake state
- The heart rate rises to near to its wakeful state
- Your limbs may even become paralyzed
- The breathing often becomes faster and even irregular

DEEP SLEEP REQUIREMENTS

While a person needs all of the sleep stages, deep sleep is particularly important for brain health and function. Deep sleep allows the brain to build and store new memories and improves its ability to collect and recall information.

This sleep stage also allows the brain to relax and recover from a day of activity, allowing it to replenish the energy for the next day in the form of glucose.

Deep sleep also plays a part in regulating hormones. During this stage, the pituitary gland secretes human growth hormone, which helps tissues grow and regenerate cells in the body.

Importantly, a person needs to get enough deep sleep to accomplish these functions. The amount of deep sleep a person has is going to contribute to how much total sleep they get. For most adults, sleeping 7-9 hours is the normal recommendation which gives the body plenty of time in the deeper sleeping conditions.

If one day the body does not get enough deep sleep, it can compensate for this the next day by moving rapidly through the cycles reach the deepest stages of sleep and remain there longer.

However, if the person does not get enough deep sleep regularly, this may begin to affect the brain.

As deep sleep plays a role in memory, if the body does not get enough sleep, it will have difficulty creating new memories or retaining the information.

How to get More Deep Sleep

There might be a few of ways to increase the amount of deep sleep a person gets every night.

As the American Sleep Association says, setting aside more time for sleep is the most important thing a person can do to increase the amount of deep sleep they get each night. Doing so helps the body to go through further stages of sleep, which promotes a deeper sleep.

Other procedures may generally help promote deep sleep and good sleep, such as:

- Exercising vigorously, such as jogging, running, or swimming early in the day rather than before bedtime.
- Make dietary changes which include fewer carbohydrates and healthy fats
- Warm up your body up in a spa or hot sauna

Additionally, some antidepressants may help people get deeper sleep, though this is not the case for everyone.

Pink noise can also make a person's deep sleep more effective. Pink noise is a random noise, with components that are more low-frequency than normal. A research in the journal Frontiers in Human

Neuroscience explored the effects on deep sleep by using sound stimulation, such as pink noise. The findings suggested that listening to these sounds could improve the deep sleep state of a person, resulting in better memory function when they wake up.

Some general healthy sleep habits can also help to promote better sleep experience, including:

- Avoid blue lights, such as computers or smartphones near bedtime
- Keep the room as quiet as possible by closing windows and turning off lights on alarm clocks
- Avoiding caffeine later in the day
- Reducing stress
- Avoiding big meals before bedtime
- Set a schedule for sleep and try to fall asleep at the same time every night

Deep sleep is an integral part of the sleep process, but it is just one component of a good night's sleep. There may be several ways to encourage deeper sleep, such as exercising or listening to pink noise while falling asleep.

The best way to get deeper sleep can be as simple as setting side enough time to sleep every night.

What Are the Benefits of Deep Sleep?

During deep sleep, the metabolism of glucose in the brain

increases, promoting short- and long-term memory and general learning.

Deep sleep is also when the pituitary gland secretes vital hormones, such as human growth hormone, contributing to growth and body development.

Other benefits of deep sleep include:

- increasing blood supply to muscles
- energy restoration
- cell regeneration
- strengthening the immune system
- promoting growth and repair of tissues and bones

What Happens When You do not get Enough Deep Sleep?

Deep sleep is responsible for helping to process the information that you come across every day. Without enough sleep, the brain cannot commit that information to your memory.

Not getting a good sleep is often related to conditions, such as:

- diabetes
- stroke
- Alzheimer's disease
- heart disease

The deep sleep stage itself is related to certain disorders, like:

- bedwetting
- sleep eating
- sleepwalking
- night terrors

How Much Deep Sleep do You Need?

You spend about 75% of your night in non-REM sleep, and the other 25% in REM sleep. Of this, deep sleep is around 13% to 23% of your total sleep.

Deep sleep diminishes with age. You have two hours of deep sleep each night if you are under 30. If, on the other hand, you are over 65, you may get just half an hour of deep sleep every night, or none at all.

Deep sleep is not necessarily needed, but younger people may need more because it encourages growth and development. Older people often need deep sleep, but not getting much does not necessarily indicate a sleep disorder.

How do You Know How Much You're Getting?

If you wake up feeling tired, this could be an indication that you haven't had enough deep sleep.

Wearable devices at home measure sleep by monitoring the changes in your body during the night. Still, this technology is relatively new. Although it can help to identify the patterns of sleep, it may not be an accurate measure of how much deep sleep you get.

Your doctor may recommend a sleep study known as Polysomnography (PSG). You'll sleep in a laboratory during this test while you're hooked up to monitors that measure:

- body movements
- heart rate
- breathing rate
- oxygen levels
- brain waves

Your doctor can use this information to see if you are reaching deep sleep and other stages throughout the night.

Tips for Better Sleep

The heat will spur more slow- wave sleep. Taking a hot bath or spending time in a sauna before bed, for example, may help improve the quality of your sleep.

Eating a low-carbohydrate diet or taking certain antidepressants may also promote deep sleep, though further research in this area is needed.

Overall, getting enough sleep can increase your deep sleep too.

Here are some tips:

- Set yourself to a bedtime routine where you go to sleep and wake up every day at the same time
- Get plenty of exercises. Every day is a good start, about 20 to

30 minutes, just stop working out in the hours before bedtime

- Stick to water and other decaffeinated drinks before bedtime. Alcohol, caffeine, and nicotine will make having a good night's rest more difficult

- Create a bedtime routine, such as reading a book or taking a bath to relax from the day

- Remove flashing lights from your bedroom and loud noises. Too much time on the TV or computer will make it difficult to relax

- Do not lie tossing and turning in bed. Try doing a light activity, such as reading, until you're exhausted again

- Consider changing your pillows if you've had them for more than a year and find it difficult to get comfortable

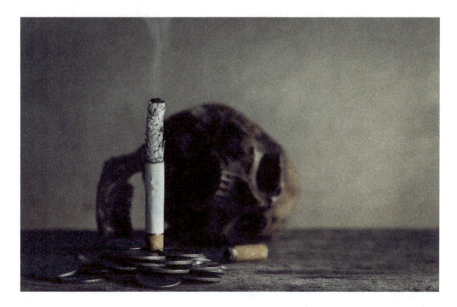

DEEP SLEEP: HOW TO GET MORE OF IT

We already know what deep sleep is, and how our bodies need it to function properly, but what exactly is it? There is a large body of deep sleep research, but we have all the knowledge we need to know about what it is, its purpose and how you can get more of it.

Deep sleep is the stage of sleep that is related to the slowest brain waves during sleep. This period of sleep is known as slow-wave sleep because the EEG activity is characterized by slow waves with a relatively high amplitude and a frequency of less than 1 Hz. A down-state implies the initial portion of the wave; an inhibition period during which the neurons in the neocortex remain silent. It is during this period that the neocortical neurons will relax.

An upstate indicates the next section of the wave; an excitation period during which the neurons fire briefly at a rapid rate. This state is a phase of depolarization, whereas the former state is a phase of hyperpolarization. In comparison to Rapid Eye Movement Sleep (REM sleep cycle), absent or slow eye movement, lack of genital activity, and moderate muscle tone are the main characteristics of slow-wave sleep.

Research Behind Sleep Stages and Deep Sleep

Deep sleep can be defined as stage three of non-rapid eye movement sleep and is often referred to as "slow-wave sleep" according to the 1968 Rechtschaffen & Kales (R & K) Standard. There is no significant distinction between stages three and four; however, stage three has delta activity of 20% to 50%, while stage four has more than 50%. The American Academy of Sleep Medicine has no longer referred to stage four since the year 2008, and stage three and four merged to create stage three. A duration of 30 seconds of sleep, consisting of 20% or more slow-wave sleep, is therefore now called stage three. One of the Stages of Sleep is slow-wave sleep (deep sleep).

Features of Deep Sleep

- High arousal threshold
- Presumed restoration of body and brain
- Electroencephalograph (EEG) demonstrates delta waves (low frequency, high amplitude)
- Consolidation of memories

Why is Deep Sleep Important?

Deep sleep is essential for consolidating new memories and is sometimes referred to as "sleep-dependent memory processing." Therefore, individuals with primary insomnia may have impaired memory consolidation and will not function as effectively as regular patients after a period of sleep. Therefore, slow-wave sleep increases the declarative memory, and this involves both episodic and semantic memory.

A core model was built on the premise that long-term memory storage is facilitated by interaction between the neocortical and hippocampal networks. Several studies indicate that there was a substantially higher density of human sleep spindles as compared to the non-learning control task until subjects were conditioned to learn a declarative memory task. It is due to unconscious wave oscillations, which make up the intracellular recordings from thalamic and cortical neurons.

Function of Deep Sleep

Studies of human sleep deprivation seem to indicate that the primary function of deep sleep may be to allow the brain time to recover from its everyday operation. The increase in the metabolism of glucose in the brain is attributed to activities involving mental activity. Another feature affected by slow-wave sleep is the release of the growth hormone, which at this point is at its highest. This also causes an increase in parasympathetic neural activity as well as a decline in sympathetic neural activity.

The highest arousal thresholds are observed in deep sleep, such as the intensity of being disturbed by the sound of a specific volume. When a person wakes up from slow-wave sleep, they are usually not very alert. Cognitive tests after awakening does indicate that mental performance can be impaired for periods of up to 30 minutes as compared to other stage awakenings. This phenomenon is called "sleep inertia."

After sleep deprivation, there is often a fast recovery of slow-wave sleep, meaning that the next bout of sleep will involve not only more slow-wave sleep than normal but deeper slow-wave sleep. In addition to the duration of sleepless period, the preceding duration of this stage will decide the duration of slow-wave sleep. The key factor to consider when determining the amount of slow-wave sleep in any given sleep period is the length of the preceding sleeplessness, which is usually correlated with the build-up of sleep-inducing substances in the brain.

Sleep Disorders During Deep Sleep

There are many sleep disorders and parasomnia that often occur during slow-wave sleep. Sleepwalking (Somnambulism), bed-wetting (Enuresis), sexsomnia, night terrors, and sleep eating are all associated with slow-wave sleep. People with narcolepsy often have fragmented deep sleep.

Factors that Increase Slow-Wave Deep Sleep

Severe prolonged exercise and body heating, such as immersion in a sauna or hot tub, are factors which have shown to improve slow-wave sleep during the sleep period that follows.

Studies have shown that slow-wave sleep is induced when the temperature of the brain reaches a certain threshold. It's believed that this threshold is regulated by circadian rhythm and homeostatic processes. An exceptionally low, short-term carbohydrates diet in healthy sleepers causes an increase in the percentage of slow-wave sleep. This involves an increase in the percentage of dreaming sleep (REM sleep) compared to a mixed diet regime. It is thought that these changes in sleep could very well be linked to the metabolism of the fat content in a low carbohydrate diet.

Additionally, ingestion of antidepressants and certain SSRI's can increase the duration of slow-wave sleep periods; however, THC's effects on slow-wave sleep remain controversial. In such cases, overall sleep time is always unchanged because of the alarm clock, circadian rhythms, or early morning commitments of a person.

How to Get More Deep Sleep

The most important thing you can do to increase your amount of deep sleep is to give yourself more total time to sleep. Individuals may also deprive themselves of complete sleep. REM sleep is also reduced, in addition to decreasing deep sleep.

Some data suggest that intense exercise can improve or stabilize deep sleep. Some sleeping specialists recommend aerobic activities such as running, swimming, and jogging. It is better for those who are prone to insomnia to work out earlier in the day and not before bedtime.

Stage three of the stages of the sleep cycle, slow-wave sleep (deep sleep), is an important part of the cognitive function. It plays an essential part in consolidating memory and rebuilding the brain. Because of its value to your overall health, you have to increase your amount of deep sleep by allowing you to have enough total nightly sleep time. In addition, exercise and a balanced diet are different approaches that you can use to help make your slow-wave sleep better.

HOW TO INCREASE DEEP SLEEP

If you find yourself having the necessary nighttime hours of sleep but still thinking your body hasn't rejuvenated itself, you probably aren't getting enough deep sleep. This stage of sleep is responsible for healing and rebuilding the body, replenishing cells and revitalizing the immune system, as opposed to light sleep. It's a critical rest stage, but we often don't get enough of it. Deep sleep will make up about 10-20 percent of your entire night's rest. The first cycle of deep sleep lasts 45 to 90 minutes, and from there each subsequent cycle gets shorter.

If you wake up feeling exhausted after 7 to 9 hours of sleep, there are a few steps you can take to improve your time in deep sleep.

HOW TO INCREASE DEEP SLEEP

- **Keep Your Diet Sleep-Friendly**

The American Sleep Association found that, relative to those who eat a mixed diet, a low carbohydrate diet causes an improvement in deep sleep time. There's also a growing body of evidence suggesting that drinking bitter cherry juice will help increase the time spent in deep sleep.

- **Try Pink Noise**

A recent Northwestern Medicine study found that pink noise, such as waves lapping on a beach or trees rustling in the wind, increased the amount of time spent in deep sleep. While it only studied 13 people, it's an exciting exploration of sleep solutions in the world. There are some great sound machines that feature every sound variety, including pink noise. Give one a try and see if your deep sleep improves.

- **Hypnosis Before Bed**

A 2014 study by the University of Fribourg in Switzerland found that subjects listening to sleep-promoting audio recordings of hypnotic suggestions spent as much as 80% more time in deep sleep compared to those not listening to the recordings. There are both free and paid audio resources offering a form of hypnosis and using one might help with your deep sleep deficit.

- **Get the Right Amount of Exercise**

The National Health Institutes suggest about 30 minutes of exercise a day, 5 days a week. That's right at the sweet spot between what's best for deep sleep enhancement and your overall sleep quality. Try not to overdo it though, too much physical activity can often lead to sleep problems or even insomnia. Try something you enjoy doing for the 30-minute average per day. Fortunately, you don't have to become a cross-country sprinter or a cross-fit junkie to work out for better sleep. Easy exercise such as walking the dog, light jogging and even yoga can do the trick as well. It takes good sleep to find the energy you need to exercise every day.

- **Listen to ASMR Videos**

Have you heard of ASMR? A 2015 study defined it as, "Autonomous Sensory Meridian Response in which individuals experience a tingling, static-like sensation across the scalp, back of the neck and at times additional areas in response to specific audio and visual stimuli. It is widely reported that this sensation is accompanied by feelings of relaxation and well-being. "This study found that 82% of respondents used ASMR to help them sleep, and 70% used it to manage stress. There's a wide number of ASMR vloggers out there, and each caters for different ASMR triggers."

You can get the deep sleep your body requires to recover your strength, muscles and physical well-being through exercise, a healthy diet and some other new tricks. Try out these ideas and see what works tonight for you!

CHAPTER 10
CALM YOUR MIND

Life constantly throws chaos at us — whether it's our relationships, our finances, or our health. In the world of work, around 50% of people are burned out in industries such as banking, and health care, and employers spend $300 billion a year on stress related issues in the workplace.

We just keep moving through, surviving on adrenaline, in response. We overschedule ourselves; we're drinking another coffee; we're responding to another post. When we stay hyperactive all the time, we believe that ultimately, we will get things done.

But all that does is burn us out, drain our productivity, and make us exhaust ourselves.

There is another way — a more relaxed way. Cultivating a more comfortable and confident state of mind does not mean we are going to sink in all of our responsibilities. Research suggests that tackling them would get us more attention, creativity, and energy, and research also points to easy ways we can tap into the peaceful state of mind in our stressful lives to be more resilient.

A STRESSED MIND VS. A CALM MIND

Stress was never meant to be a 24/7 experience. As Stanford professor Robert Sapolsky states, in the five minutes just before you die, you are just expected to feel depressed. If a wild animal chases you in the savanna, your reaction to stress is supposed to save your life — it mobilizes your energy, your muscles and your immune system to get you out of danger quickly. When animals flee, they come into the "rest-and-digest" state after the fight-or-flight state, where the parasympathetic nervous system is working to replenish their energy.

The stress response should be short-lived because it is wearing down your body, health and energy. It also influences things like your emotional outlook and the way you make decisions. You are more likely to react to situations when you are stressed than to answer with reason.

You perceive the world differently, too. Stress makes us fractious, and we cannot see the bigger picture. Our focus gets wider when we're calmer, we really see more things. Participants in one study completed a three-month meditation session.

They then engaged in something called the attentional blink task, in which you watch photos appear quickly one after the other. If people do this exercise, their mind usually doesn't pick up all the target pictures. However, after the training in meditation, participants were able to pick up more of the target images than pre-treatment — suggesting their state of mind had become more attentive.

Being able to show greater attention means you know more about other people and can interact more easily with them. For an evolutionary reason, high stress and anxiety (or any form of negative emotion) make us self-focused: when our ancestors were stressed, it was because they were in a situation of survival. It was good to concentrate on yourself, so you can save your life.

If we're stressed, we're less likely to notice if a friend looks burned out or depressed, and more likely to get annoyed if they're not doing as we expect. But when you're in a calmer and happier place, it's probably the day you're going to have more empathy: you're going to notice your colleague and take the time to reach out and ask if you can do anything to support them.

You can control your energy when you are calm because you are not constantly burning yourself out, spending your days in overdrive with your sympathetic nervous system. Calm lets you concentrate on what you need to do and get it done quickly.

Calmness can also influence your creativity. Research shows that when we're not actively concentrating or stressed, our most creative thoughts come in moments. When our brain is in alpha wave mode, which is a relaxed state of mind, we are at our most creative — like when you are in the shower or taking a stroll in nature. People who go four days on an immersive nature retreat come back with creativity increased by 50 percent.

If you want to make the most of yourself in terms of productivity, innovation, and creativity — making progress at work or just addressing the simple life issues you face — calm is the key.

How to Cultivate a Calm State of Mind

We do know how to get stressed. Many of us are excellent at stimulating and overloading our adrenal system. The problem then is, how do you wind down? Research suggests some behaviors that not only feel good but also place us in a calmer, more comfortable state — a state from which we are better able to cope with whatever life throws at us.

1. Breathing

Jake, who appears in the book The Happiness Track, was an American Marine officer in charge of a Humvee on a convoy through Afghanistan, as he was driving his vehicle passed over an improvised explosive device. He looked down after the blast and found his legs badly broken below the knee. In that moment of surprise, panic and pain, he recalled a breathing exercise he had read about for situations of intense wartime.

It allowed him to fulfil his duty, which was to inspect everyone else in the vehicle. It gave him the presence of mind to issue instructions for help, and then to tourniquet his own legs and support them until he fell unconscious — that saved his life.

Our breathing is an effective way of controlling our emotions and we take it for granted. Through your breath, you can activate your parasympathetic nervous system -the calming response in your body.

That's why we switched to breathing to help veterans—50% of whom see little improvement from therapy or treatment for their trauma symptoms. The veterans were doubtful but we started teaching them various exercises in breathing. Some of them began sleeping without medication within a couple of days; after the week-long program, many of them no longer qualified as having post-traumatic stress, and that persisted until a year later.

You can change how you feel by using your breathing. Researchers observed people experiencing various emotions in another study, and noticed there was a different breathing pattern for each. We then gave the various breathing patterns to other people to follow, and asked them, "How do you feel? "It turned out that relaxation exercises actually evoked the emotions.

One of the most calming breathing exercises you can do is breathe in (for example, to a count of four), hold and then breathe out for up to twice as long (for example, to a count of six or eight). You should gently close your mouth, making a sound like the ocean, which is used to breathe deep relaxation. As you do this, especially thanks to those long exhalations you stimulate the parasympathetic nervous system, reducing your blood pressure and heart rate.

2. Self-compassion

We are our worst critic. We claim that being self-critical can help us become more self-conscious and make us work harder, but this is a fallacy. Indeed, according to much study, self-criticism is undermining our resilience. When we criticize ourselves , we are less likely to learn from our mistakes. Self-critical people tend to be more depressed and anxious, and unable to bounce back from the struggles.

Imagine someone running a marathon in their life for the very first time, and they trip and fall. On the sidelines, someone says, "You are a loser, you are not a runner. What is it you are doing here? Go home. "That person is the voice of our inner self-criticism. On the other hand, self-compassion is someone who says, "everybody falls, that's normal. You are so amazing; you are absolutely killing this.

Self-compassion is the ability to be mindful of your emotions — conscious of the emotions going on inside if you fail at anything. It doesn't mean you identify with them; you can simply watch them and note them without feeding the flames. Self-compassion also involves understanding that mistakes are made by everyone and that it is part of being human. And, it's the opportunity to say to yourself exactly the way you'd speak to a friend who failed, kindly and warmly.

Research shows that when we follow this way of thinking, we are calmer — we have less feelings of tension and lower levels of cortisol. We're much more resilient: We're less afraid of failure and more motivated to get better.

3. **Connection**

How often are we really 100% there for another person? When

was the last time anyone, including your partner, was 100 percent there with you?

There is an epidemic of loneliness in the USA and around the world. We know these feelings of loneliness are extremely destructive to our mind and body, leading to poorer health and even earlier death. The tensions and lack of peace in the world today can add to this loneliness because of the way it tends to make us self-centered.

After food and shelter, our greatest human need is to connect with others in a positive way. We have a deep and profound desire to belong to one another from the moment we are born until our last day. And when we meet that need, it brings us calm: The oxytocin and natural opioids we release when we connect can exert a calming influence on our bodies, and the knowledge that we have the support of others can soothe our minds. Research suggests that when we face adversity, our relationships and our community have a part to play in our resilience.

So how do we build a state of mind where we feel more connected?

The good news is that you can turn your focus outward and feel more connected by taking care of yourself and your own well-being through activities such as breathing and self-compassion. Positive feelings such as calm, of course, help us feel closer to others. You may also try different practices that research has found to improve your sense of connection.

4. Compassion for others

Imagine a day where things will not go well for you — you have spilled your coffee on yourself, and it's raining, and then a friend calls who has a real problem in their life, and you get up and go quickly to help them. What's happens to your state of mind in that moment?

All of a sudden, you have a lot of energy; you are at their disposal. That's what practicing compassion, altruism, and service does to your life.

It increases your well-being tremendously as many of us have experienced little acts of kindness when we act in this way. Our heart rate goes down when we feel compassion and our parasympathetic nervous system gets more activated.

Compassion and kindness can help to protect us from adversity as well. Researchers have found in one of my favorite studies that people who had endured stressful life situations had a shorter lifespan.

But there was a small group of people among those participants who just seemed to keep on living. What'd happened to these people?

When the researchers dug a little deeper, they found that they were all involved in helping friends and relatives in their lives — from assisting with transportation or shopping to housework and child care. Service is one of the deepest ways of nurturing the community around you but also of nurturing, inspiring and energizing yourself. It's like that children's book — when you fill somebody's bucket, it fills up yours too.

Cultivating calmness is not about suppressing all kinds of unpleasant emotions. In fact, when we make time to breathe, connect and care, some of the negative feelings we've been running from could catch up with us. But this is the time of self-compassion; it is all right to feel bad. Resilience doesn't mean we're going to be happy all the time, but it does mean we have the mindset, the energy, and other people's support to help us weather the storm.

CHAPTER 11
HOW QUITTING SMOKING HAS CHANGED MY LIFE

Years of smoking ingrains behaviors and patterns of thought which are more about addiction than our true feelings and preferences.

Once we stop smoking, we are often surprised at changes in attitude toward smoking and life in general.

Steve, a member of DelphiForums About Smoking Cessation support group, recently gathered some new (and some not-so-new) ex-smokers to discuss how smoking cessation has changed their way of thinking and acting.

Their responses are posted below; But first, the question from Steve and then a glimpse into how smoking cessation impacts our lives positively.

From Steve:

"When we smoked, we had a certain mentality. When we quit and obtained our freedom from addiction, our mentality changed. What's the biggest change or transformation in thought that you've experienced since you quit smoking?"

Transformations Brought on By Quitting

- "After I quit, I began to understand how much I really didn't like it! I haven't become that bad an ex-smoker, but give me a couple more years!" ~ Steve

- "At the end of 10 months, I am now more optimistic and more careful in my thinking. When I make a decision, I take my time to think about all the possibilities. I feel better in my resolve to stay a non-smoker, as well. It amazes me how proud I am of my ability to finally feel that I will remain a non-smoker. I never really believed I could do this after 44 years of smoking. My thinking has been changed forever." ~Deb

- "I think I'm more concerned about myself now: my health, I'm standing up for myself when necessary, I feel like there are more possibilities out there without my smoking monkey on my back." ~ Linda

- "I learned that I don't need cigarettes to know when I'm sad, happy, anxious, bored, stressed, surprised, angry, impatient, nervous, confused, scared, lost, or any other emotion. The only thing I did was to temporarily reduce the symptoms of withdrawal from nicotine and hide my emotions behind a veil of smoke." ~Jenn

- "I'm now a different person than I was on Feb. 28, 2013. I'm more aware of what I'm eating since I quit smoking. I lead a healthier lifestyle. I'm a more kind, thoughtful, and patient person than when I was smoking. I like who I've become rather than the person who was ruled by a cigarette ... I'm so happy to be on the other side ... I'm happy." ~Gail

- "The reality checks after I read on the NRT patches that patch exposure can destroy small household pets and kids. Something so deadly, without even a flame, blows my mind. When I walk or walk around the property, I'm taking small trash bags with me now to try to clean up after litterers (straw as well as cigarette butts). It's amazing how throwing a filter into water can kill a fish, a salamander, and other small aquatic wildlife. When I'm feeling healthy and can get out and about, I guess I have kind of made it my mission to stop others from hurting wildlife that did not choose to smoke or come into contact with poison." ~Rose

- "I've been leading a busy life. I've never had time to smoke because of all the smoke time I wanted. Now, I can "do" stuff, and I don't have to sit down and smoke away while I think about it. I still delay to some extent ... but it's a lot better." ~Vivienne

- "Quitting smoking changed me in a lot of ways, but I believe the enhanced empathy, the willingness to put myself in someone else's shoes was a big one. One of my favorite quotes from Maya Angelou is proven day after day: "I've learned that people will forget what you've said, people will forget what you've done, but people can never forget how you've made them" ~Dee

- "I'm a new quitter. I've been nicotine-free for 24 days! I've noticed changes in my outlook in this short time. I find myself more confident —- like if I can quit smoking, I can accomplish other things I may have thought impossible! This fresh feeling is a lovely and unexpected surprise." ~Mmac

- "I've walked through so many transformations in the past [smoke-free] 8 months, and I'm sure I'm going to keep changing a few more times, but today I feel confident in myself, and I feel grateful for finding such a great group of people to get me here. The anger, fear, and confusion I had at the beginning of my journey is gone-Hallelujah!" ~Peggy

- "I think one improvement for me was seeking comfort in solitude. Instead of taking drags on a cigarette, I'm enjoying the peace and relaxation of deep breaths. I'm seeing clearly instead of a cloud of smoke, and I've gained more patience." ~Andrea

- "The change seems to be evolving for me. I guess this evolution first became apparent to me about the sixth months after quitting smoking. I suddenly wasn't depressed anymore, and I figured this was because my brain had adjusted for the first time in 35 years to have a normal dopamine level."

- "The second indication of the change was when I discovered that I could get a level of inner peace when I breathed deeply at around the tenth month, and it's getting better. I never felt better, physically in my life. I don't want to sound too arrogant, but I can't even look at a pack of cigs anymore without seeing them as a poison I don't want to have any part of."

- "But I want to stay on this journey more than anything else to see how much better it can actually get." ~Rick

As smokers, most of us feel that stopping smoking makes life dull and less satisfying. Cigarettes are with us all day, every day. The idea that we do not have them triggers fear in our hearts.

The truth of life without smoke is quite the opposite. When we start overcoming nicotine addiction, the benefits that we didn't expect start showing, and we can settle comfortably into our new lives. It doesn't happen immediately, but it will happen if you allow yourself the time and space required to recover from this addiction

Do not let fear of life stop you from getting started with smoking cessation. The benefits shot outweigh the discomforts.

TOM USED HYPNOSIS TO STOP SMOKING

I really wanted to quit smoking, but I couldn't.

I smoked for twenty years, starting my late teens, which I now remember as especially stupid because I was a competitive athlete (in soccer) at the time I started my habit. I have taught abroad for most of my adult life, and many of the countries I lived in (especially parts of Europe and Asia) were more open to public smoking than America is. When I returned home, I found that I was no longer able to smoke in restaurants, in homes of other people, and in other places where I had become used to lighting up, and I felt alone. Smoking has always aggravated my asthma, and I knew of course that it's very deadly too. But I just couldn't stop.

I have tried cold turkey (which worked several times, once for two years), nicotine gum, wellbutrin, and a nicotine patch to quit in the past. And about six months ago, I was on depression and alcohol abuse treatment, and my doctor suggested attempting to stop smoking using therapeutic hypnosis. As I decided to stay away from some sort of chemical treatment (such as anti-depressants, or even therapies based on nicotine), I was interested. I kind of felt like, why not?

I found hypnosis surprisingly accessible, and not weird. This felt to me like a combination of a relaxation treatment and a counseling session. I felt very relaxed but not "out of it," as in movies. I felt that I was present. I think that's helped cut me down. I haven't stopped, just about half of what I used to smoke. Smoking to me now is not an automatic response. Hypnosis seems to have made me calmer, or at least more aware that I have a choice.

I found my hypnotherapist through my counselor on chemical addictions. I don't know if my psychologist, or my regular doctor who I see for asthma, would have suggested hypnosis. However, they did not speak out against it. I guess they're just glad to see people trying to stop smoking in whatever way they can!

I felt that some people thought it was strange, a kind of "magical thinking," but none of my practitioners advised against it, and most people were really interested in knowing more about it once you started talking about it.

I'd say hypnosis isn't for everybody, but it's definitely worth trying. I know it can't hurt, and really could help, so why not? I feel the same about other holistic therapies: when I was in Asia, I tried acupuncture and massage therapy, and both helped me with various health issues, including asthma to anxiety

CONCLUSION

Smoking cigarettes is the greatest single cause of illness and premature death in the US. The number is far bigger worldwide. Every year, tobacco kills about seven million people, although about one million deaths are due to exposure to second-hand smoke by non-smokers.

Although nearly 80,000 people in the US die each year from smoking-related illnesses, one in five adults are still regular smokers.

Now things appear to be changing. Forty years ago, 51 percent of males and 41 percent of females were smokers. Those rates have dropped by more than half, with 15% of adults in the U.S. smoking, and 59% claiming they never smoked.

Quitting smoking is one of the biggest challenges a person faces, and often they need more than just willpower. A lot of options are available now; from campaigns like Stoptober and local community groups to medications. Hypnotherapy provides an attractive solution for many people.

Self-hypnosis can be used to help you achieve meaningful changes in your life, such as stopping smoking. Find your session time and place – make sure it's quiet enough so you won't be interrupted.

Lie or sit down and close your eyes. Take three slow, deep breaths, keep the third breath in for three seconds. Then as you breathe out, relax and sink back into your seat. Focus on your breathing, and let your thoughts flow in and out as if attached to your breath until you have cleared your mind.

Now count backwards from 10 to 0, counting each number as you breathe out and focusing on another area of your body, enabling it to relax. I begin with my toes and work up to my head, but you can try head down to your feet, you prefer to do so. Whichever works.

You're going to be relaxed at this point, but to help deepen that relaxation, imagine yourself in a quiet place. I like using the beach: Picture the beach in as much detail as possible. If you hate beaches, try to imagine a meadow or garden, wherever you feel most relaxed.

Now you are in that state of concentration and relaxation; you can make a suggestion to yourself, feel more confident about quitting smoking, or visualize your reason for quitting more vividly so that you feel increasing motivation to achieve your goal. It is your time, so make wise use of it.

Once it's time to wake up, just count yourself back from 0 all the way up to ten and you will find yourself wide awake, feeling refreshed and re-energized. If for whatever reason, you need to be fully awake and ready during your session, you're going to be, and can automatically bring yourself awake. That's it! It's really that easy to start making meaningful life changes."

If you enjoyed this book, please let me know your thoughts by leaving a short review on Audible... Thank you

CPSIA information can be obtained
at www.ICGtesting.com
Printed in the USA
LVHW010149220221
679513LV00003B/317